Wall Pilates Workouts for Women:

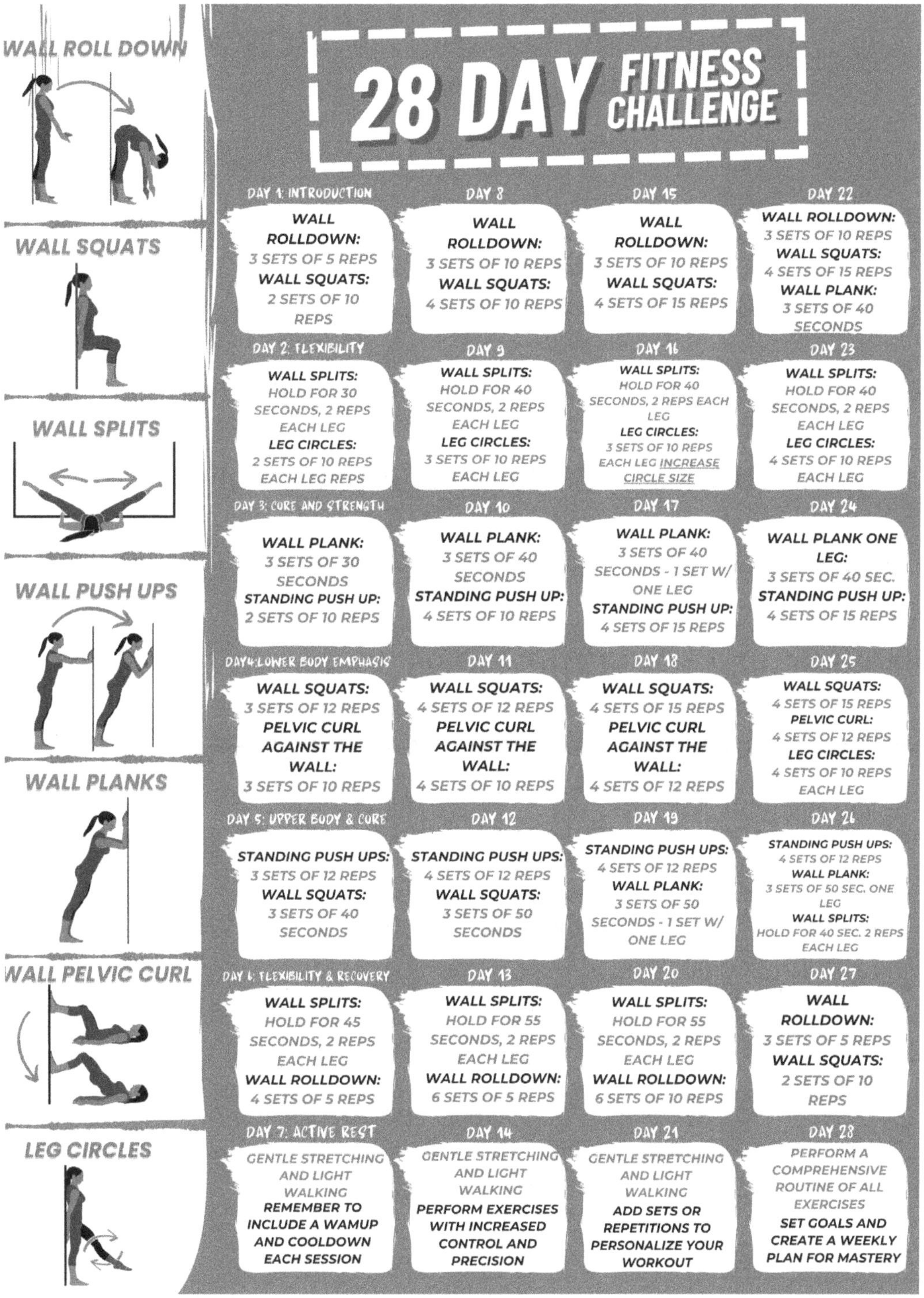

WALL ROLL DOWN

WALL SQUATS

WALL SPLITS

WALL PUSH UPS

WALL PLANKS

WALL PELVIC CURL

LEG CIRCLES

28 DAY FITNESS CHALLENGE

DAY 1: INTRODUCTION
WALL ROLLDOWN: 3 SETS OF 5 REPS
WALL SQUATS: 2 SETS OF 10 REPS

DAY 2: FLEXIBILITY
WALL SPLITS: HOLD FOR 30 SECONDS, 2 REPS EACH LEG
LEG CIRCLES: 2 SETS OF 10 REPS EACH LEG REPS

DAY 3: CORE AND STRENGTH
WALL PLANK: 3 SETS OF 30 SECONDS
STANDING PUSH UP: 2 SETS OF 10 REPS

DAY 4: LOWER BODY EMPHASIS
WALL SQUATS: 3 SETS OF 12 REPS
PELVIC CURL AGAINST THE WALL: 3 SETS OF 10 REPS

DAY 5: UPPER BODY & CORE
STANDING PUSH UPS: 3 SETS OF 12 REPS
WALL SQUATS: 3 SETS OF 40 SECONDS

DAY 6: FLEXIBILITY & RECOVERY
WALL SPLITS: HOLD FOR 45 SECONDS, 2 REPS EACH LEG
WALL ROLLDOWN: 4 SETS OF 5 REPS

DAY 7: ACTIVE REST
GENTLE STRETCHING AND LIGHT WALKING
REMEMBER TO INCLUDE A WAMUP AND COOLDOWN EACH SESSION

DAY 8
WALL ROLLDOWN: 3 SETS OF 10 REPS
WALL SQUATS: 4 SETS OF 10 REPS

DAY 9
WALL SPLITS: HOLD FOR 40 SECONDS, 2 REPS EACH LEG
LEG CIRCLES: 3 SETS OF 10 REPS EACH LEG

DAY 10
WALL PLANK: 3 SETS OF 40 SECONDS
STANDING PUSH UP: 4 SETS OF 10 REPS

DAY 11
WALL SQUATS: 4 SETS OF 12 REPS
PELVIC CURL AGAINST THE WALL: 4 SETS OF 10 REPS

DAY 12
STANDING PUSH UPS: 4 SETS OF 12 REPS
WALL SQUATS: 3 SETS OF 50 SECONDS

DAY 13
WALL SPLITS: HOLD FOR 55 SECONDS, 2 REPS EACH LEG
WALL ROLLDOWN: 6 SETS OF 5 REPS

DAY 14
GENTLE STRETCHING AND LIGHT WALKING
PERFORM EXERCISES WITH INCREASED CONTROL AND PRECISION

DAY 15
WALL ROLLDOWN: 3 SETS OF 10 REPS
WALL SQUATS: 4 SETS OF 15 REPS

DAY 16
WALL SPLITS: HOLD FOR 40 SECONDS, 2 REPS EACH LEG
LEG CIRCLES: 3 SETS OF 10 REPS EACH LEG _INCREASE CIRCLE SIZE_

DAY 17
WALL PLANK: 3 SETS OF 40 SECONDS - 1 SET W/ ONE LEG
STANDING PUSH UP: 4 SETS OF 15 REPS

DAY 18
WALL SQUATS: 4 SETS OF 15 REPS
PELVIC CURL AGAINST THE WALL: 4 SETS OF 12 REPS

DAY 19
STANDING PUSH UPS: 4 SETS OF 12 REPS
WALL PLANK: 3 SETS OF 50 SECONDS - 1 SET W/ ONE LEG

DAY 20
WALL SPLITS: HOLD FOR 55 SECONDS, 2 REPS EACH LEG
WALL ROLLDOWN: 6 SETS OF 10 REPS

DAY 21
GENTLE STRETCHING AND LIGHT WALKING
ADD SETS OR REPETITIONS TO PERSONALIZE YOUR WORKOUT

DAY 22
WALL ROLLDOWN: 3 SETS OF 10 REPS
WALL SQUATS: 4 SETS OF 15 REPS
WALL PLANK: 3 SETS OF 40 SECONDS

DAY 23
WALL SPLITS: HOLD FOR 40 SECONDS, 2 REPS EACH LEG
LEG CIRCLES: 4 SETS OF 10 REPS EACH LEG

DAY 24
WALL PLANK ONE LEG: 3 SETS OF 40 SEC.
STANDING PUSH UP: 4 SETS OF 15 REPS

DAY 25
WALL SQUATS: 4 SETS OF 15 REPS
PELVIC CURL: 4 SETS OF 12 REPS
LEG CIRCLES: 4 SETS OF 10 REPS EACH LEG

DAY 26
STANDING PUSH UPS: 4 SETS OF 12 REPS
WALL PLANK: 3 SETS OF 50 SEC. ONE LEG
WALL SPLITS: HOLD FOR 40 SEC. 2 REPS EACH LEG

DAY 27
WALL ROLLDOWN: 3 SETS OF 5 REPS
WALL SQUATS: 2 SETS OF 10 REPS

DAY 28
PERFORM A COMPREHENSIVE ROUTINE OF ALL EXERCISES
SET GOALS AND CREATE A WEEKLY PLAN FOR MASTERY

Table of Contents

28-Day Fitness Challenge from Beginner to Advanced Increase Circulation, Reduce Muscle Cramps & Improve Digestion and Sleep

Hey there! I'm thrilled to have you join me on this exciting journey. You've heard of Pilates, and perhaps you've even tried it. Pilates, with its focus on core strength, flexibility, and overall body awareness, has been transforming bodies and minds for years. But have you ever heard of Wall Pilates?

Why Wall Pilates, you may ask? Well, it's a fantastic variation of traditional Pilates that utilizes the wall as a prop to deepen stretches, enhance stability, and increase the challenge level of specific exercises. It's a unique twist that adds a whole new dimension to the practice.

Now, I need to let you in on a little secret: Pilates, especially Wall Pilates, is not just a fitness regimen; but a journey. A journey that everyone, regardless of age, gender, or fitness level, can embark on. It's not about perfection; it's about progress. So, Wall Pilates is for you whether you're a seasoned athlete, a busy mom, or simply someone looking to improve your health and wellness.

In this book, we will walk this fitness journey together. Your path to health and well-being is tailored to your individual needs and goals. Through practical advice, detailed exercises, and motivational insights, we'll explore how Wall Pilates can transform not just your body but your mind too.

Remember, it's not just about the destination; it's about the journey. Let's get started on yours. Welcome to Wall Pilates Workouts for Women: 28-Day Fitness Challenge from Beginner to Advanced in order to Increase Circulation, Reduce Muscle Cramps & Improve Digestion and Sleep.

Chapter 1: The Impact of Wall Pilates on Overall Health and Wellbeing

Do you remember the last time you felt truly balanced? Picture yourself standing tall, both physically and emotionally and mentally. Wouldn't it be remarkable if we could capture that feeling and make it part of our everyday lives? That's where Wall Pilates comes in. This innovative fitness practice, which uses a wall as a prop, is a game-changer in the world of health and fitness. It's not just about looking good; it's about feeling good from the inside out.

Let's get down to the specifics. We'll begin by exploring the physical benefits of Wall Pilates and understand how it can significantly improve your posture, flexibility, and core strength.

The Gift of Good Posture: Stand Tall with Wall Pilates

Good posture is more than just standing tall; it's about aligning your body to reduce strain on your muscles and joints. Poor posture can lead to a host of problems, including back pain, neck strain, and even breathing difficulties.

Enter Wall Pilates. One of the core principles of Pilates is alignment, and by using the wall as a prop, you can get immediate feedback on your posture. The wall serves as a guide, helping you align your head, shoulders, and hips in a straight line. Over time, this practice can help correct imbalances and promote better posture.

Consider the Wall Roll Down, a simple yet effective exercise. By standing against the wall and slowly rolling down vertebra by vertebra, you're working your core and learning to maintain spinal alignment. It's like having a personal trainer at your disposal, guiding you to hold your body in the correct posture.

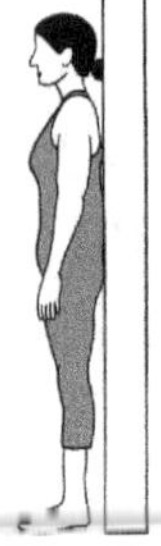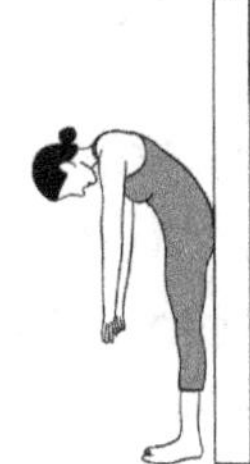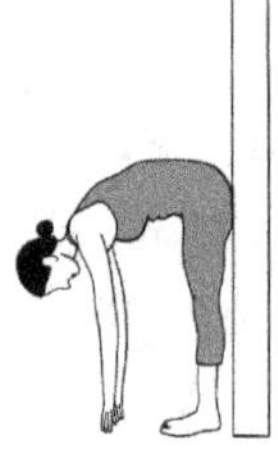

5Embrace Flexibility: Stretch and Lengthen Your Body

Flexibility is often overlooked in fitness routines, but it's key to maintaining a healthy and functional body. It allows us to easily perform daily activities and reduces the risk of injuries.

Wall Pilates, with its emphasis on controlled, flowing movements, is a fantastic way to enhance flexibility. The wall provides the support you need to stretch your muscles to their full range of motion safely.

Unlock Your Core Power: Strengthen from Within

We're not just referring to flat abs when we talk about core strength. The core is your body's powerhouse, including your abdominal muscles, lower back, pelvis, and hips. A strong core enhances balance, stabilizes your body, and allows you to perform physical activities with greater ease.

Wall Pilates is a core-centric workout. Almost every move you perform against the wall engages your core muscles. **The Wall Plank,** for instance, is an excellent exercise that targets your entire core. It's more challenging than a traditional plank as the wall adds an element of instability, forcing your core to work harder to maintain balance.

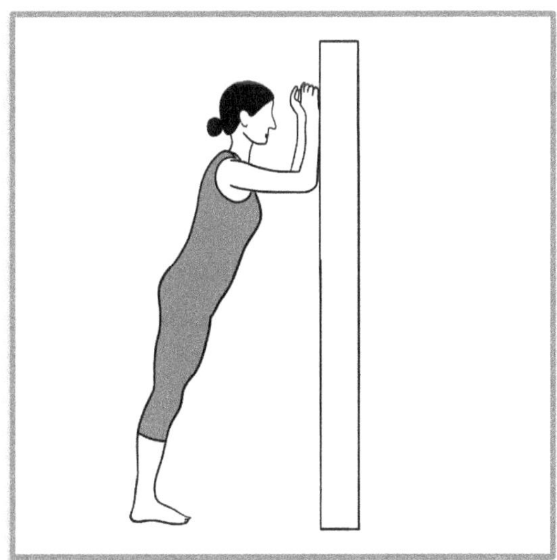

But here's the best part: the stronger your core, the better your overall performance in Wall Pilates and other physical activities. It's a virtuous cycle of fitness!

In essence, Wall Pilates is a gateway to a healthier, stronger, and more balanced body. It's a practice that challenges, supports, and rewards you with visible and tangible benefits. But remember, everybody and every Wall Pilates journey is unique. Embrace the process, listen to your body, and most importantly, enjoy every moment. Your path to better health and well-being begins here. One Wall Pilates move at a time.

Mental Health Advantages: More Than Just a Workout

Stress Reduction: The Calm Amidst Life's Storms

We all know life can get hectic. Deadlines, family commitments, endless to-do lists - it's easy to feel overwhelmed. Here's where Wall Pilates shines as a beacon of calm. This practice invites you to slow down, breathe, and reconnect with your body. Each exercise requires focus and precision, allowing you to quiet your mind and temporarily set aside your worries. You're in a safe space, your very own sanctuary of tranquillity.

Let's take a moment to visualize the Wall Roll Down exercise. As you stand against the wall, you're asked to tune into your breath and gradually roll down, vertebra by vertebra. It's a soothing rhythm, almost meditative. With each exhale, you release tension; with each inhale, you draw in calmness. By the end of your session, you're not just physically refreshed; you're mentally rejuvenated too.

Enhanced Focus and Concentration: Harnessing the Power of the Present

In today's fast-paced world, our attention is often pulled in a hundred different directions. The constant bombardment of information can leave us feeling scattered and mentally fatigued. Enter Wall Pilates, a practice that encourages you to cultivate focus and heighten your awareness.

Consider the Wall Plank exercise. It's a move that demands your complete attention. You need to align your body correctly, engage your core, and maintain balance - all while breathing steadily. There's no room for your mind to wander. As you hold the plank, you're fully present, immersed in the moment. It's an exercise in mindfulness, a skill that extends beyond the mat and into your daily life. Regular practice can sharpen your concentration, boost your productivity, and improve your mental clarity.

Improved Mood: The Joy of Movement

Imagine waking up on a grey, gloomy morning. You're feeling sluggish, maybe a little down. Now, picture yourself rolling out your mat, standing next to your wall, and starting your Wall Pilates routine. You can feel your energy levels rising with each stretch and controlled movement. By the time you're done, you're not just wide awake; you're brimming with positivity.

This isn't just a scenario; it's backed by science. Physical activity triggers the release of endorphins, the body's natural feel-good hormones. Wall Pilates, with its combination of stretching, strengthening, and controlled breathing, is an exceptional mood booster. It's a practice that brings joy, uplifts your spirits, and infuses positivity into your day. So, the next time you're feeling low, remember: your wall, your mat, and a good mood are just a Pilates session away.

Our minds and bodies are intricately connected, and Wall Pilates beautifully highlights this bond. It's not just about building a stronger body; it's about fostering a healthier mind. It's an invitation to slow down, tune in, and truly experience the joy of movement. With Wall Pilates, fitness becomes a celebration of what your body can do and how it can make you feel. So, step onto your mat, lean into your wall, and let the transformation begin.

Wall Pilates and Long-Term Health:

Keeping Injuries at Bay: The Proactive Approach
Wall Pilates is not just about the 'now'. It's a fitness practice that looks ahead, planning for a future where your body continues to serve you well. When it comes to injuries, prevention is better than cure, and Wall Pilates is a proactive measure you can take.

The wall, steadfast and supportive, is an excellent training tool. It provides the stability needed for safe and effective exercise, making it less likely for injuries to occur. Take, for instance, the **Wall Squat.** This exercise strengthens the muscles of your lower body, but with the added support of the wall, it's kinder on your joints, reducing the risk of knee injuries.

Moreover, the focus on alignment and balanced muscle development in Wall Pilates helps prevent injuries that can arise from muscular imbalances or poor posture. It's like having an invisible shield safeguarding your body as you move through life's various stages.

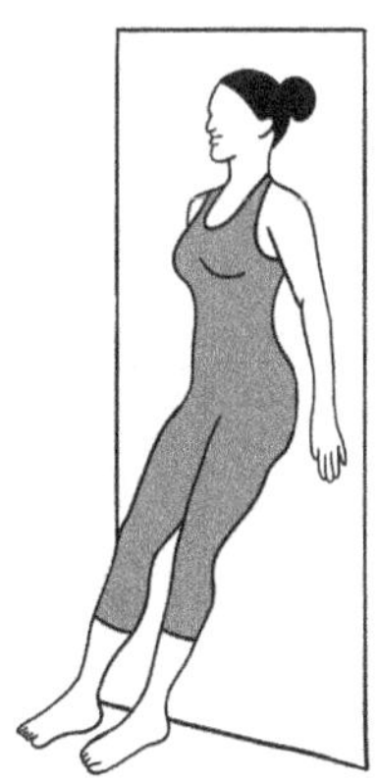 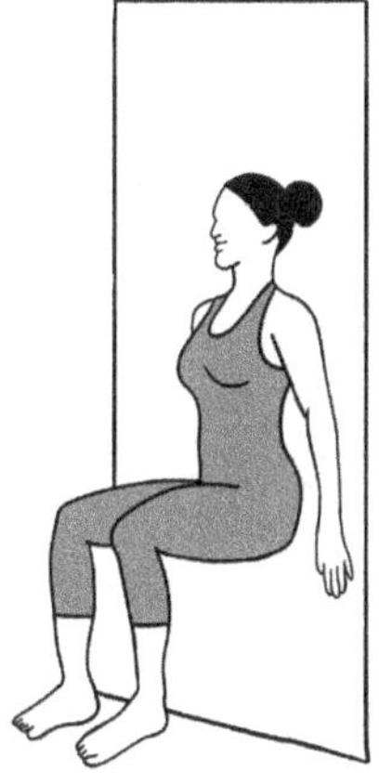

Cardiovascular Health: A Heart-Friendly Workout

When we think of cardio, we often picture high-intensity workouts that leave us breathless. But cardiovascular health isn't just about running marathons or doing intense activity sessions. It's about keeping our hearts in good shape by engaging in regular, moderate-intensity exercise.

Wall Pilates, while not a typical cardio workout, can contribute to a healthy heart. The controlled movements and mindful breathing can elevate your heart rate into the moderate-intensity range. This is particularly true for exercises that engage large muscle groups, such as the Wall Mountain Climbers or the Wall Plank Jacks. These exercises get your heart pumping and blood flowing, contributing to better cardiovascular health.

Strong Bones, Strong Body: The Role of Weight-Bearing Exercise
Did you know that our bones, like muscles, respond to exercise by becoming stronger? Weight-bearing exercises, where you work against gravity, are particularly beneficial for bone health. They stimulate bone-forming cells and help prevent bone loss as we age.

Wall Pilates is an excellent form of weight-bearing exercise. Many of the exercises, such as the Wall Push-Up or the Wall Plank, draw on your body weight for resistance. As you push against the wall, your bones are subjected to a healthy amount of stress, which encourages them to become stronger. It's like a mini workout for your bones, helping to maintain their density and strength.

Wall Pilates is more than a workout; it's a commitment to long-term health. It's about keeping injuries at bay, nurturing a healthy heart, and building strong bones. It's a practice that equips you with the strength and resilience needed to enjoy a fulfilling, active life.

Pilates, The Wall, and You: A Recipe for Lifelong Health
Wall Pilates is not a quick fix; it's a lifestyle choice. It's about making a commitment to your health today so you can reap the benefits tomorrow and for years to come. And the beauty of it is it's accessible to everyone. All you need is a wall, a mat, and a willingness to embrace the practice.

So, let's make that commitment together. Let's discover the power of Wall Pilates, not just as a path to a fitter body but as a way to better health and well-being. Let's build strength, enhance flexibility, improve posture, reduce stress, and nourish our minds and bodies. Let's make Wall Pilates a part of our lives for life.

The Future is Bright: Your Wall Pilates Journey Begins Now

So, are you ready to embrace Wall Pilates? Remember, this is your journey. It's not about perfection; it's about progress. It's about learning to love and respect your body, challenging yourself, and enjoying every step of the process. Your path to health, flexibility, and core power begins here. Let's get started!

Real Stories of Transformation: The Power of Wall Pilates in Everyday Lives
Now that we've explored the numerous benefits of Wall Pilates let's turn our attention to some real-life transformations. These are not tales of overnight success; they are stories of persistence, dedication, and the transformative power of Wall Pilates. These individuals have embraced the practice, made it a part of their lives, and reaped the rewards. Let's hear their voices.

First, let's meet Lisa, a busy mother of two. Juggling work and family life left her with little time for fitness. She was constantly tired, her posture was starting to slump, and she longed for a change. That's when she discovered Wall Pilates.

Lisa shares, "I was immediately drawn to Wall Pilates for its convenience. I didn't need any fancy equipment - just a wall. I started with just 15 minutes a day, and within weeks, I was feeling stronger and more energized. My posture improved, and I found myself standing taller. But the best part? I was doing something for myself, and that felt wonderful."

Next, we have Mike, an avid runner. Despite being fit, he often struggled with tight muscles and occasional back pain. Upon a friend's recommendation, he decided to give Wall Pilates a try.

Mike reflects, "I was skeptical at first. But as I got into it, I began to appreciate the focus on flexibility and core strength. I found my running performance improving and my muscle soreness reducing. Wall Pilates has now become a staple in my fitness routine."

Let's move on to some detailed case studies that illustrate the effectiveness of Wall Pilates. Karen, a 45-year-old office worker, had been struggling with chronic neck pain due to long hours at the computer. Regular physiotherapy sessions provided temporary relief but didn't address the root cause - her poor posture.

Karen recalls, "I was desperate for a solution. I started Wall Pilates and was amazed at the focus on alignment and posture. The wall helped me understand where my body should be in space. Over time, my neck pain diminished, and I felt more confident and comfortable in my body. Wall Pilates was a lifesaver."

Another case is Tom, a retired 65-year-old man who was looking for a low-impact exercise routine to stay active. He discovered Wall Pilates and was drawn to its focus on balance and stability, crucial aspects of fitness as we age.

Tom shares, "Wall Pilates has been incredible. My balance has improved, I feel stronger, and I love how the exercises are easy on my joints. It's a workout I look forward to, and it's significantly impacted my health and quality of life."

There's also Alex, a former professional athlete. After a career-ending injury, he was left feeling lost. Wall Pilates helped him regain his strength, recover his confidence, and even find a new career path as a Pilates instructor.

Alex says, "Wall Pilates gave me a second chance. It helped me rehabilitate my body and redefine my identity beyond sports. Now, as an instructor, I get to share the benefits of Wall Pilates with others. It's been a truly transformative journey."

Finally, meet Sarah, a woman who turned her life around with Wall Pilates. Struggling with obesity and low self-esteem, she was searching for a fitness routine that she could stick to. Wall Pilates entered her life at the right time.

Sarah recounts, "Wall Pilates was a revelation. The exercises were challenging but doable, and I could modify them to suit my level. I started noticing changes - not just physical, but also mental. I was happier, more confident, and most importantly, I felt strong. I've lost weight, but more than that, I've gained a love for movement and an appreciation for my body."

These stories illuminate the power of Wall Pilates to transform lives. They remind us that fitness is not just about physical strength but mental resilience, self-love, and the courage to embrace change. So, as you step onto your mat and lean into your wall, remember: each stretch, each breath, each moment is a step towards your own transformation.

Chapter 2: Unraveling the Threads of Time: The History of Pilates

Have you ever wondered about the origins of the exercises you perform against your wall? Each movement, each position, is a piece of a story that spans over a century, a story that begins with a visionary named Joseph Pilates. Join me as we step back in time and explore the birth of Pilates, a fitness revolution that continues to inspire and transform lives across the globe.

The Birth of Pilates
Joseph Pilates and His Vision

Born in Germany in 1883, Joseph Pilates was a frail child suffering from asthma, rickets, and rheumatic fever. Determined to overcome his physical limitations, he immersed himself in the study of anatomy and Eastern and Western forms of exercise, including yoga, martial arts, weightlifting, and gymnastics.

As he experimented with these disciplines, Joseph developed a unique approach to physical fitness, one that emphasized the integration of mind, body, and spirit. He believed that physical health was the first requisite of happiness and stressed the importance of 'contrology' or control, a concept that remains central to Pilates today.

His vision was to create a fitness system that enhanced overall health, improved posture, and cultivated a balanced body and mind. Although the term "Pilates" would not be used until after his death, the foundation for this transformative practice was laid by Joseph Pilates himself.

The Original Pilates Studio

Fast forward to the 1920s. Joseph Pilates had moved to New York and opened his fitness studio, attracting a diverse clientele, including dancers, actors, and athletes. His studio, fitted with unique apparatuses designed to support and challenge the body, became the birthplace of the Pilates method.

Joseph and his wife Clara, a trained nurse, taught their students exercises that promoted strength, flexibility, and balanced muscle development. They emphasized precision, control, and smooth, flowing movements, principles that continue to define Pilates today.

The exercises were performed on specially designed equipment, including the Reformer, a sliding carriage device, and the Cadillac, a raised platform with a variety of attachments. Joseph also developed mat exercises that required no equipment, paving the way for the accessibility of Pilates as we know it today.

Pilates During the War Years

During World War I, Joseph Pilates was interned as an "enemy alien" in Britain. Despite the challenging circumstances, he continued to refine his fitness approach. He began training his fellow internees, helping them maintain their health and strength within the confines of the internment camp.

During this time, Joseph started experimenting with springs attached to hospital beds, aiming to assist bedridden patients with their exercises. This innovation marked the early development of the Pilates Reformer, a key piece of equipment in contemporary Pilates studios.

These years also witnessed the remarkable effect of the Pilates method on overall health. It was reported that none of Joseph's trainees succumbed to the 1918 flu pandemic, a testament to the power of his holistic fitness approach.

From the humble beginnings in a small German town to the bustling studios in New York, the journey of Pilates is a testament to the vision and tenacity of Joseph Pilates. His dedication to physical health and wellness laid the foundation for a fitness revolution that continues to thrive over a century later.

The birth of Pilates is more than a historical event; it's the spark that ignited a global movement. It's the seed from which grew a tree of knowledge, a tree whose branches extend into our homes, guiding and supporting us as we practice Wall Pilates. As we delve deeper into the history of Pilates, we'll discover how this tree continues to grow and evolve, reaching new heights and spreading its roots into diverse fields of health and wellness. So, let's continue our journey through time, exploring the evolution of Pilates and its impact on the world of fitness.

Pilates in the Modern World and the Fitness Boom

In the late 20th century, the world began to witness a surge in health consciousness. As people became more mindful of their well-being, the fitness industry flourished. Amid this revolution, Pilates emerged as a beacon of holistic fitness, harmonizing the physical and the mental, the strength and the flexibility, the exertion and the relaxation.

The modern fitness landscape, with its focus on low-impact, whole-body workouts, was a fertile ground for Pilates to thrive. Its unique blend of strength, flexibility, and mindfulness resonated with fitness enthusiasts searching for an exercise regimen that catered to their body, mind, and spirit. Suddenly, Pilates was not just a niche workout but a global fitness trend.

Gyms and wellness centers around the world began to introduce Pilates classes, incorporating the innovative exercises designed by Joseph Pilates into their routines. The Reformer, once a unique feature of Pilates studios, found its way into mainstream gyms. Mat Pilates classes started popping up everywhere, from local community centers to upscale fitness clubs. Pilates had truly arrived on the global fitness stage.

Pilates and Rehabilitation

As Pilates continued to gain popularity, another interesting trend emerged. Health professionals, particularly physiotherapists, began to recognize the potential of Pilates in injury rehabilitation. Its emphasis on controlled movement, core strength, and improved flexibility made it an ideal therapy for a variety of ailments.

Pilates proved to be particularly effective in rehabilitating back injuries. Its focus on core strength and spinal alignment helped alleviate back pain, improve posture, and enhance overall back health. Physiotherapy clinics began to incorporate Pilates exercises into their treatment plans, helping patients regain strength, improve mobility, and accelerate their recovery.

But the rehabilitation benefits of Pilates didn't stop at physical injuries. Its mindful, meditative aspect was found to be beneficial in managing stress and reducing anxiety. Mental health professionals started recommending Pilates as a complementary therapy, helping patients find balance and tranquility amid their mental health struggles. Pilates was now a fitness routine and a pathway to holistic healing.

The Global Spread of Pilates

The turn of the century marked a significant milestone in the Pilates story. The Pilates method, once confined to a small studio in New York, had spread its wings and taken flight across the globe. It had transcended cultural boundaries, resonating with people from diverse backgrounds and lifestyles.

In Europe, Pilates became a staple in wellness retreats and fitness resorts, attracting health tourists with its promise of a rejuvenating mind-body workout. It found a harmonious blend in Asia with traditional practices like yoga and tai chi, creating a fusion of Eastern and Western philosophies. Down under in Australia, Pilates studios started dotting the sunny coasts, offering beachgoers a different kind of wave to ride.

Armed with their mats and Reformers, Pilates instructors travelled far and wide, bringing Joseph Pilates' vision to life in corners of the world he could have only dreamed of. They adapted and evolved the Pilates method, tailoring it to their communities' unique needs and cultures. From bustling cities to serene villages, from the young to the old, from the athlete to the office worker, Pilates has become a global fitness phenomenon, touching and transforming lives one workout at a time.

The story of Pilates in the modern world is a testament to its timeless appeal and universal relevance. It's a narrative of how a humble fitness method born in a small German town could become a global wellness revolution. It's a reminder that good health, just like Pilates, knows no boundaries or limits. As we move forward, let's take a moment to marvel at the remarkable journey of Pilates, celebrating its past even as we look forward to its future.

The Invention and Rise of Wall Pilates
The Genesis of Wall Pilates

In the late 20th century, the principles of Pilates branched off into a unique form known as Wall Pilates. As the name suggests, this discipline involves using a wall as a prop to enhance the effectiveness of traditional Pilates exercises. But who came up with this ingenious idea?

The concept was born out of a simple observation: not everyone has access to specialized Pilates equipment like the Reformer or Cadillac, but almost everyone has access to a wall. Fitness enthusiasts started experimenting with exercises against the wall, discovering its potential to intensify workouts and stretches.

A single person did not invent Wall Pilates; rather, it evolved organically within the Pilates community. It was a response to a need for more accessible and affordable Pilates workouts. It embodied the spirit of innovation and adaptability, traits that are at the heart of the Pilates philosophy.

Wall Pilates and Home Fitness
The emergence of Wall Pilates coincided with a growing trend towards home fitness. As people sought ways to stay fit within the comfort of their homes, they discovered the practicality and versatility of Wall Pilates.

The wall served multiple purposes: it was a support system, a tool for balance, a surface for resistance, and an aid for alignment. Exercises such as the Wall Roll Down, Wall Push-Up, and Wall Plank became popular choices for home workouts. They were easy to learn, required no equipment, and could be modified according to individual fitness levels.

Wall Pilates was a home workout and a solution to common fitness challenges. It addressed the issue of space constraints, allowing people to exercise effectively in small apartments or studios. It provided a means to maintain consistency, enabling individuals to stick to their workout routines despite busy schedules or changing circumstances. In essence, Wall Pilates brought the benefits of a Pilates studio into the household, making it a pivotal player in the home fitness movement.

The Growing Popularity of Wall Pilates

With its practicality and effectiveness, it was no surprise that Wall Pilates quickly gained popularity. Fitness enthusiasts embraced the concept, valuing its simplicity and convenience. They found that they could get a comprehensive workout, targeting various muscle groups and improving overall fitness, just by using a wall.

The rise of digital media further propelled the popularity of Wall Pilates. Fitness instructors started sharing Wall Pilates routines on social media platforms and YouTube, reaching a global audience. People from different parts of the world, regardless of their fitness backgrounds, started practicing Wall Pilates. They discovered a community of like-minded individuals, all united by their love for this unique form of exercise.

The popularity of Wall Pilates also caught the attention of health and wellness professionals. Physiotherapists recognized its potential as a therapeutic exercise, particularly for improving posture and enhancing balance. Psychologists appreciated its mindfulness aspect, noting its potential to reduce stress and improve mental well-being.

From its humble beginnings as a home workout to its global recognition as a comprehensive fitness practice, the rise of Wall Pilates has been nothing short of remarkable. It has shown us that fitness is not bound by the confines of a gym or the limitations of equipment. It has reminded us that a wall, an everyday feature of our lives, can be an extraordinary tool for health and wellness.

The story of Wall Pilates is still being written, with each one of us contributing a chapter. As we practice our Wall Rolls and Wall Planks, we're strengthening our bodies and shaping the future of this innovative fitness discipline. And who knows? One day, our own Wall Pilates stories will become a part of this fascinating history.

Technological Advances and Pilates

In a rapidly advancing world of technology, it's hard not to see its influence on how we work out. For Pilates, technology has been a powerful ally, opening up new possibilities and shaping the future of the practice.

Virtual reality, for instance, is making waves in the Pilates world. Imagine donning a VR headset and finding yourself in a serene Pilates studio, complete with an instructor guiding you through your workout. You could be in your living room, but it feels like you're in a tranquil oasis, immersed in your Pilates routine.

There's also the rise of fitness apps and online platforms, providing access to Pilates workouts at the touch of a button. These digital tools allow you to practice Pilates anytime, anywhere, breaking down barriers of time and location. They offer a variety of workouts, catering to different fitness levels and personal preferences, making Pilates more accessible than ever before.

Wearable technology, like smartwatches and fitness trackers, is adding another dimension to Pilates practice. These devices can monitor your heart rate, track your calories, and even provide feedback on your form. They bring a level of precision and personalization to your workouts, helping you get the most out of your Pilates sessions.

Pilates and Holistic Health Trends

Broader trends in the health and wellness industry are also shaping the future of Pilates. There's a growing shift towards a more holistic approach to health, where physical fitness is just one part of the equation.

This aligns perfectly with the philosophy of Pilates, which emphasizes the integration of mind, body, and spirit. As more people seek balanced lifestyles, Pilates, with its focus on mindful movement and whole-body health, is poised to meet this demand.

Wellness retreats are incorporating Pilates into their programs, offering a blend of physical exercise, mindfulness practices, and healthy eating. Corporate wellness programs are introducing Pilates classes to their employees, recognizing its potential to reduce stress and improve productivity. Even schools are exploring Pilates, tapping into its benefits for mental focus and physical fitness among students.

The connection between Pilates and holistic health is not a new trend; it's a return to the roots. It's a reaffirmation of Joseph Pilates' original vision of a workout that nurtures the body, mind, and spirit.

The Next Generation of Pilates Practitioners

Looking ahead, the future of Pilates will be shaped by the next generation of practitioners. These are individuals who grew up with Pilates and witnessed its evolution from a niche workout to a global fitness trend.

This new generation is pushing the boundaries of Pilates, bringing fresh perspectives and creative ideas to the practice. They're blending Pilates with other fitness disciplines, infusing it with dance, yoga, or functional training elements. They're exploring new spaces for Pilates, taking it out of the studio and into the outdoors, the beach, or the office.

But more than innovation, the next generation is carrying forward the legacy of Pilates. They're upholding its core principles, maintaining its focus on quality of movement, and preserving its commitment to holistic health. They're ensuring that Pilates remains true to its roots, even as it branches out into new directions.

The future of Pilates is a tapestry woven with threads of technology, holistic health trends, and the energy of the next generation. Its future promises to be as dynamic and transformative as the practice itself.

As we close this chapter, let's carry with us the rich history of Pilates, the lessons from its past, and the promise of its future. Let's remember that our Wall Pilates practice is part of a larger story, a story that continues to unfold with each passing day. As we turn the page, let's look forward to exploring the principles that make Pilates the powerful practice it is today.

Chapter 3: Mastering the Core Principles of Pilates

Close your eyes for a moment, take a deep breath in, hold it, and then let it out slowly. What did you feel? A sense of calm? A moment of peace? That, my friend, is the power of breath - a power central to Pilates' practice. Now, let's explore how this seemingly simple act of breathing transforms your Pilates experience, and why it is more significant than you might think.

The Power of Breath Control

We often do breathing without much thought – an automatic, rhythmic process that keeps us alive. However, in Pilates, it takes center stage. Breathing in Pilates is intentional and mindful, designed to enhance your movement, focus your mind, and energize your body.

Each movement synchronises with your breath when you perform a Pilates exercise. Think of your breath as the rhythm to which your body dances. For example, while performing a Wall Roll Down, you inhale as you start the roll down, filling your lungs with oxygen, and exhale as you roll back up, releasing tension. This mindful coordination of breath with movement enhances the flow of the exercise, making it more effective and enjoyable.

Techniques for Effective Breath Control

In Pilates, we use a technique known as lateral or rib cage breathing. Imagine your torso is a balloon. As you inhale, you expand the balloon sideways, allowing your rib cage to widen. You deflate the balloon as you exhale, drawing your ribs back in. This type of breathing keeps your core engaged, which is crucial for stability and balance in Pilates.

Here's a simple exercise to practice lateral breathing. Stand with your back against a wall, placing your hands on your rib cage. Take a deep breath in, feeling your ribs expand into your hands. As you exhale, feel your ribs contract, moving away from your hands. Practice this a few times, focusing on keeping your belly still as you breathe.

The Benefits of Proper Breathing

Mindful breathing in Pilates offers a host of benefits. Firstly, it improves oxygen flow to your muscles, giving them the fuel they need to perform. This means you can do exercises more efficiently and for longer periods.

Secondly, coordinating your breath with movement helps you maintain a steady rhythm, making your workout more fluid and graceful. It's like a dance - your breath sets the tempo, and your body follows the beat.

Thirdly, focused breathing helps clear your mind, reducing stress and enhancing your overall Pilates experience. It's a moment of mindfulness, a break from the hustle and bustle of daily life. It's just you, your breath, and your body moving in harmony.

Breathing is not just a physical act; it's a holistic experience that intertwines the physical, mental, and emotional. It's a reminder that simple things often hold the most power in Pilates and life. So, the next time you lean into your wall for a Pilates workout, remember to breathe - not just because you have to, but because you recognize and appreciate the immense value it brings to your practice.

Centering: The Heart of Pilates. The Concept of the "Powerhouse"

In the language of Pilates, the term "powerhouse" holds a special significance. It doesn't refer to a single muscle or body part. Instead, think of it as your body's command center - a collective term for the group of muscles around your center, namely your abdomen, lower back, hips, and buttocks. This area is the primary source of your body's power, stability, and energy in Pilates.

Imagine you're about to perform a Wall Push-Up. Before you start, you focus on your powerhouse. You engage your abdominal muscles, align your spine, and stabilize your hips. As you move through the exercise, it's your powerhouse that supports and controls your movement. It's the anchor that keeps you grounded and the engine that drives your motion.

Techniques for Achieving Centering

The ability to tap into your powerhouse doesn't come naturally. It requires practice, awareness, and a few handy techniques:

1. Engaging your core: Before you start an exercise, take a moment to engage your core muscles. Imagine pulling your belly button towards your spine. This simple action activates your powerhouse, prepping it for the workout ahead.

2. Aligning your body: Proper alignment is central to engaging your powerhouse effectively. Ensure that your head, shoulders, and hips are in line. For instance, when performing a Wall Plank, check that your body forms a straight line from your head to your heels.

3. Breathing mindfully: Remember the power of breath? It plays a crucial role in centering as well. As you inhale, visualize your breath filling your powerhouse. As you exhale, imagine your powerhouse becoming more stable and grounded.

4. Staying focused: Keep your attention on your powerhouse throughout your workout. Even as you move different parts of your body, your focus should remain on your center.

The Impact of Centering on Performance

Centering does more than give you a good workout. It has a profound impact on your Pilates performance:

1. Increased stability: A strong, engaged powerhouse provides stability as you move, making your movements more controlled and precise.

2. Improved balance: Your powerhouse is your body's balance point. Focusing on your centre improves your balance and coordination, which is essential for advanced Pilates exercises.

3. Enhanced strength: The powerhouse is the source of all movement in Pilates. The more you engage your powerhouse, the stronger you become.

4. Greater efficiency: When you move from your center, your movements become more efficient. You use less energy to do more.

5. Reduced risk of injury: Centering promotes proper alignment and balanced muscle use, reducing the risk of injuries.

6. Better overall performance: Ultimately, centering improves your overall Pilates performance. It's the key to mastering the exercises, progressing in your practice, and reaping the full benefits of Pilates.

Centering is not an isolated aspect of Pilates. It's intertwined with every breath you take, every move you make. It's a constant practice, a conscious choice. And it's one that can transform your Wall Pilates experience, making it more powerful, more beneficial, and more rewarding. So, as you stand against your wall, ready to start your workout, remember to center. Engage your powerhouse, align your body, breathe mindfully, and stay focused. Your Wall Pilates practice starts here, in your center.

The Value of Flow in Movement: The Principle of Fluidity in Pilates

Imagine a river, its waters moving smoothly and continuously, flowing from one point to another with grace and ease. Now, picture your body moving in a similar manner during a Pilates exercise, transitioning seamlessly from one move to another. This concept of uninterrupted, smooth movement is integral to Pilates and is known as flow.

Flow in Pilates goes beyond physical movement; it's an expression of the harmony between your body and mind. It's about creating a rhythm that guides your workout, making each movement feel natural and effortless. It's about connecting each exercise, each breath, and each moment, transforming your workout into a fluid dance of strength and flexibility.

Techniques for Achieving Flow

Achieving flow in Pilates requires practice, awareness, and a few key techniques:

1. Understanding the exercise sequence: Each Pilates workout follows a specific sequence of exercises. Understanding this sequence allows you to anticipate the next move, allowing smoother transitions.

2. Using your breath: Your breath is a powerful tool for achieving flow. Coordinate your breath with your movements, using your inhales and exhales to guide your transitions.

3. Maintaining focus: Keep your attention on your body and the movement at hand. This mental focus will help you move more controlled and fluidly.

4. Practicing regularly: Like any skill, achieving flow takes practice. The more you perform a sequence of exercises, the more naturally you'll be able to flow from one move to another.

The Benefits of Smooth, Flowing Movements

1. Efficiency: Flow allows you to move more efficiently during your workout. By seamlessly transitioning from one exercise to the next, you're able to maintain your rhythm and momentum, making your workout more effective.

2. Grace and Agility: Flowing movements help to develop grace and agility. They enhance your coordination, balance, and flexibility, which can improve your performance in other physical activities.

3. Mindfulness: Flowing movements encourage mindfulness. As you focus on moving with control and precision, you become more in tune with your body, enhancing the mind-body connection.

4. Enjoyment: Let's not forget enjoyment. Flowing movements make your Pilates workout more enjoyable. As you move with fluidity and grace, you'll find yourself immersed in the experience, making your workout more engaging and fulfilling.

The principle of flow is a beautiful aspect of Pilates, bringing a sense of grace, continuity, and enjoyment to your workout. It's a reminder that Pilates is more than a series of exercises; it's a dance of strength, flexibility, and control. So, next time you're practicing Wall Pilates, remember to find your flow. Let your movements be smooth and continuous, let your breath guide you, and let yourself enjoy the dance.

The Mind-Body Connection in Pilates

In Pilates, your mind is just as engaged as your body. This mind-body practice requires concentration, mindfulness, and a deep awareness of your body's movements. This focus enhances your workout, promotes mental clarity, and reduces stress.

Concentration in Pilates is about being fully present in the moment. It's about tuning into your body, noticing how it feels and how it moves. It's about listening to your breath, sensing its rhythm, and coordinating it with your movements. It's about quieting the mind and focusing on the here and now.

Techniques for Enhancing Mind-Body Awareness

1. Body Scanning: Before starting your workout, take a few moments to scan your body. Notice any areas of tension or discomfort and make a mental note to move those areas gently.

2. Mindful Breathing: Use your breath to enhance your mind-body connection. As you inhale, imagine your breath reaching every part of your body. As you exhale, envision any tension or stress leaving your body.

3. Visual Imagery: Use visual imagery to enhance your movements. For example, when performing a Wall Roll Down, imagine your spine as a string of pearls, each pearl slowly lowering towards the ground.

4. Quiet Environment: Create a quiet, peaceful environment for your Pilates practice. This will help you tune out distractions and focus on your workout.

The Benefits of a Strong Mind-Body Connection

1. Improved Performance: Being mindful of your movements can improve your Pilates performance. You'll be able to move with more precision, control, and efficiency.

2. Injury Prevention: By tuning into your body, you'll be more aware of your limits, helping to prevent injuries.

3. Stress Reduction: Focusing on your body and breath can help reduce stress and promote relaxation.

4. Enhanced Wellbeing: Overall, a strong mind-body connection can enhance your sense of well-being. You'll feel more in tune with your body, more present in the moment, and more peaceful in your mind.

The mind-body connection is a fundamental aspect of Pilates, reminding us that our mental and physical health are intertwined. As you practice Wall Pilates, remember to be mindful, to concentrate, and to listen to your body. Your Pilates practice is a time to reconnect with your body, to appreciate its strength and flexibility, and to celebrate its ability to move, breathe, and flow.

The Role of Concentration in Pilates

In your Pilates practice, your brain is just as engaged as your body. The act of concentrating on each movement, each breath, and each moment is a key factor in the effectiveness of your workout. Concentration in Pilates is about being fully present, fully engaged, and fully aware. It's about moving with intention, tuning into your body and its signals, and connecting with your inner strength.

Picture yourself preparing for a Wall Plank. Before you even start to move, you're concentrating. You're focusing on your alignment, engaging your core, and preparing your mind for the task ahead. As you move into the plank, your concentration intensifies. You're aware of every muscle contraction, every breath, and every sensation. This deep, focused concentration turns a physical exercise into a holistic mind-body practice.

The Benefits of a Strong Mind-Body Connection

1. Enhanced Performance: When you're fully present and focused on your workout, you're more likely to perform each exercise correctly and efficiently.

2. Injury Prevention: Being aware of your body can help you avoid injury. You'll be more likely to notice if something doesn't feel right, allowing you to adjust your form or take a break if needed.

3. Greater Enjoyment: When you're fully engaged in your workout, you're more likely to enjoy it. You'll feel more connected to the practice, which can make your workouts more satisfying and rewarding.

4. Stress Reduction: Focusing on your body and breathing can help you tune out distractions and reduce stress. It's a chance to put aside your worries and just be present in the moment.

5. Improved Mental Wellbeing: Regular mindfulness practice, like the kind you get in Pilates, has been linked to improved mental well-being. It can help reduce anxiety, improve mood, and enhance overall quality of life.

6. So, the next time you roll out your mat for a Wall Pilates workout, remember to engage your mind as well as your body. Focus on your movements, breathe with intention, and stay present in the moment. By strengthening your mind-body connection, you'll enhance your Pilates practice and cultivate a sense of balance and harmony that extends beyond the mat.

Chapter 4: Unveiling the Truth: Debunking Wall Pilates Myths and Misconceptions

Imagine you're at a party, and someone mentions they've started doing wall Pilates. Immediately, a flurry of comments erupts. "Isn't that just for women?" someone asks. "But doesn't it cause injuries?" another person adds. "I heard it's not really a workout," someone else chimes in. Suddenly, wall Pilates, a practice you've come to love and appreciate, is shrouded in myths and misconceptions. It's time to set the record straight.

Tackling Common Misconceptions
Debunking the "No Pain, No Gain" Myth

We've all heard it before - the age-old saying, "No pain, no gain". It's a phrase that has been ingrained in our fitness culture, leading many to believe that if a workout doesn't hurt, it's not effective. But is there truth in this statement? Let's dissect it.

Pilates, including wall Pilates, operates on a different principle. It's about moving with control and precision, not pushing your body to the point of pain. While you might feel a burn as your muscles work, you should never experience pain during or after a Pilates session. In fact, regular Pilates practice can help alleviate chronic pain, particularly in the lower back, by promoting better posture and core strength.

So, the next time you're doing a wall Pilates workout, remember that pain is not a measure of effectiveness. Listen to your body, respect its limits, and strive for progress, not pain.

Addressing Fears of Injury

Injury fears often crop up when discussing any form of exercise, and wall Pilates is no exception. "Won't I hurt myself doing those moves?" is a common concern. It's a valid question, but it's one that's rooted more in fear than fact.

One of the primary aims of Pilates is to enhance body awareness. This means you become more attuned to your body, its capabilities, and its limitations. You learn to move in a way that respects and protects your body, reducing the risk of injury.

Wall Pilates, in particular, is designed with safety in mind. The wall provides support and stability, allowing you to perform exercises with correct form and control. Of course, like any exercise regimen, the risk of injury exists if exercises are performed incorrectly. That's why it's crucial to learn the proper techniques, listen to your body, and progress at your own pace.

Remember, the wall is not just a prop; it's your partner. It's there to support, guide, and help you move confidently. With the right approach and mindset, wall Pilates can be a safe and beneficial practice for individuals of all fitness levels.

Clarifying the Role of Flexibility in Pilates

"I can't do Pilates because I'm not flexible enough." Sound familiar? This is a common misconception that deters many people from trying Pilates. The truth is, you don't need to be a contortionist to practice Pilates. In fact, Pilates can help you become more flexible.

Flexibility is not a prerequisite for Pilates; it's a benefit. Pilates exercises, including those performed using the wall, incorporate dynamic stretching. This means you're gradually increasing your range of motion and flexibility as you practice.

Think of the Wall Roll Down. As you roll down, vertebra by vertebra, you're gently stretching your spine and the back of your body. With regular practice, you can roll a little bit further, reach a little bit lower, and move a little bit easier.

So, if you're hesitating to try wall Pilates because you can't touch your toes, don't worry. Pilates meets you where you are and helps you improve from there. It's not about how flexible you are; it's about improving your body's function and flexibility through consistent practice.

Conclusion

Myths and misconceptions are part of the fitness world, and wall Pilates is no exception. But by understanding the truth about this practice, we can appreciate its benefits and potential. Wall Pilates is not about pain, it's not a high-risk activity, and it's certainly not limited to those who are flexible. It's a practice that is accessible, safe, and beneficial for everyone. So, let's shed these misconceptions and embrace the truth: Wall Pilates is for all bodies, all levels, and all people. Let's celebrate this practice for what it is - a pathway to strength, flexibility, and overall wellness.

Discussing the Ideal Frequency of Workouts

Now that we understand the significance of the core, let's tackle another common query: "How often should I practice Wall Pilates?"

The answer is not one-size-fits-all. It depends on various factors, including your fitness level, goals, schedule, and other physical activities. However, as a guideline, aiming for two to three sessions per week is a good starting point.

Why this frequency? Wall Pilates is designed to be a low-impact yet effective workout. This means it can be practiced regularly without putting excessive strain on your muscles and joints. Doing two to three sessions a week allows you to consistently engage and challenge your muscles, leading to improvements in strength, flexibility, and overall fitness.

But remember, this is just a guideline. Listen to your body. Some weeks, you might feel energetic and motivated to do more. In other weeks, you might need extra rest and recovery. That's perfectly okay. Consistency is key in wall Pilates, but so is flexibility and self-care.

Addressing Concerns About Age and Fitness Level
Often, people wonder if age or fitness level can be a barrier to practicing wall Pilates. The short answer? Absolutely not!

Wall Pilates is an inclusive practice designed for everybody and every body. Whether you're in your 20s or 60s, a seasoned athlete or a fitness newbie, wall Pilates has something to offer you.

For the younger crowd or those with a solid fitness base, wall Pilates can serve as a powerful tool to enhance strength, flexibility, and endurance. It can complement other physical activities, improve sports performance, and aid in injury prevention.

Wall Pilates can provide a safe, low-impact workout for older adults or those just starting on their fitness journey. It can help improve balance, promote better posture, increase mobility, and enhance overall health and well-being.

The beauty of wall Pilates lies in its adaptability. Exercises can be modified or advanced to suit your individual needs and abilities. The wall provides a stable and supportive prop, accommodating a range of fitness levels.

So, don't let age or fitness level hold you back. Wall Pilates is not about how old you are or how fit you are. It's about moving your body, challenging yourself, and, most importantly, enjoying the process. It's a practice that embraces diversity, encourages progression, and celebrates every small victory along the way.

In the world of wall Pilates, every age is the right age, and every level is the perfect level. All you need to start is a wall, a mat, and a willingness to try. So, here's an invitation: join the wall Pilates community. Your body will thank you, and your future self will too.

Clarifying the Do's and Don'ts of Wall Pilates

In the fascinating world of wall Pilates, there are certain guidelines that can make your practice more effective, enjoyable, and, most importantly, safe. Just as a painter needs to understand the basics of brush and canvas to create a masterpiece, a Pilates practitioner needs to master the fundamentals to reap the full benefits of the practice. Let's explore these do's and don'ts, starting with the importance of proper form and technique.

Proper Form and Technique: The Blueprint of Success
Think of your body as a sophisticated machine. All its parts must work together harmoniously for it to function optimally. This harmonious function is achieved in wall Pilates through proper form and technique.

Form refers to the alignment of your body during each exercise. Imagine a straight line running from the crown of your head to your heels. This line should remain unbroken throughout your practice, irrespective of whether you're doing a Wall Roll Down or a Wall Plank. It ensures that your body is correctly positioned, reducing the risk of strain and injury.

Technique, on the other hand, refers to the way you execute each movement. It involves engaging the correct muscles, coordinating your breath with your movements, and maintaining control and precision.

A simple tip to ensure proper form and technique is to visualize each movement before you perform it. See yourself moving with grace and control, maintaining your alignment, and engaging the right muscles. This mental rehearsal can greatly enhance your physical performance, making your workout more effective and safe.

Importance of Warm-Up and Cool-Down: The Bookends of Your Workout

Just as a car needs to warm up before hitting the highway, your body needs to prepare itself before diving into a Pilates workout. This preparation phase, known as the warm-up, is crucial for a safe and effective workout.

A warm-up gently increases your heart rate, warms your muscles, and primes your body for the workout ahead. It can be as simple as marching in place, doing a few shoulder rolls, or performing some light stretches.

At the other end of your workout is the cool-down phase. This is a time to gradually lower your heart rate, relax your muscles, and return your body to its resting state. It could involve a series of stretches, some deep breathing exercises, or simply lying still and allowing your body to rest.

Both the warm-up and cool-down are non-negotiable parts of your wall Pilates practice. They enhance your performance, reduce the risk of injuries, and make your workout experience more enjoyable.

Tips for Safe and Effective Workouts: Navigating the Wall Pilates Landscape

Navigating the wall Pilates landscape can feel like an adventure filled with excitement and challenges. To make this adventure safe and rewarding, here are a few tips to keep in mind:

1. Listen to Your Body: Your body is always communicating with you. Pay attention to its signals. If a movement causes pain or discomfort, stop and adjust your form or try a modification.

2. Quality Over Quantity: In wall Pilates, how you perform an exercise is more important than how many repetitions you do. Focus on doing each rep with control and precision rather than rushing through the movements.

3. Stay Hydrated: Hydration is key to a safe workout. Drink plenty of water before, during, and after your workout to keep your body hydrated and energized.

4. Use a Mat: While the wall is your primary prop in wall Pilates, a mat is also important. It provides cushioning for your body and prevents slipping during your workout.

5. Wear Comfortable Clothing: Opt for comfortable clothing that allows easy movement. Avoid loose or baggy clothes that could interfere with your workout.

6. Consistency is Key: Consistency is crucial for progress in wall Pilates. Aim to practice regularly, even if it's just for a few minutes each day.

Remember, wall Pilates is a journey of exploration and discovery. It's about understanding your body, pushing your limits, and celebrating your progress. With these guidelines in mind, you're well-equipped to navigate this journey safely and effectively, making the most of each step along the way.

Addressing the "Pilates is Only for Women" Myth

Let's kick off this section by tackling a long-standing myth about Pilates - that it's a women-only workout. Now, it's true that Pilates classes often see more female participants, and historical pictures of Pilates sessions largely feature women. However, the belief that Pilates is only for women couldn't be further from the truth.

Firstly, it's important to remember that Joseph Pilates, the founder of this practice, was a man. He developed this method for women and everyone, regardless of gender. His vision was to create a fitness system that enhanced overall health, improved posture, and cultivated a balanced body and mind for all.

Wall Pilates, like all forms of Pilates, offers benefits that are universal. It strengthens the core, improves flexibility, enhances body awareness, and promotes mind-body connection. These benefits are not gender-specific; they apply to everyone.

So, gentlemen, don't be deterred by the misconception that Pilates is a female-dominated field. Wall Pilates is an excellent addition to anyone's fitness routine, male or female. It's about time we move beyond gender stereotypes in fitness and celebrate the inclusivity and diversity that Pilates embodies.

Debunking the "Pilates is Easy" Misconception

Next, let's address a common misunderstanding about Pilates - that it's an easy or light workout. If you've ever heard someone say, "Pilates is easy, it's just stretching," you're not alone. But anyone who has experienced the burn of a Wall Plank or the challenge of a Wall Mountain Climber knows this is far from the truth.

Pilates, particularly Wall Pilates, is a full-body workout that engages multiple muscle groups simultaneously. It combines strength training, flexibility work, and balance exercises. It requires mental focus, physical stamina, and controlled, precise movements. To put it simply, Pilates is anything but easy.

However, it's essential to understand that Pilates is not about pushing your body to extreme limits. It's not a workout to leave you breathless and sweaty. Instead,

Pilates is about controlled, mindful movement. It's about quality over quantity, precision over power. It's a workout that challenges you but in a different way than a high-intensity cardio session or a heavy weightlifting workout.

So, the next time you hear someone dismiss Pilates as easy, invite them to try a Wall Pilates workout. They might be surprised to discover the strength, control, and focus it requires.

Clarifying the Role of Pilates in Weight Loss

Finally, let's discuss a topic that often comes up in fitness conversations: weight loss. Many people wonder, "Will Pilates help me lose weight?" The answer is not as straightforward as you might think.

Firstly, it's important to remember that weight loss is a complex process influenced by many factors, including diet, physical activity, sleep, stress levels, and genetics. Exercise, including Pilates, is just one piece of the weight loss puzzle.

That being said, Pilates can contribute to weight loss in several ways. It's a physical activity that burns calories, though not as many as high-intensity workouts like running or cycling. More importantly, Pilates helps build lean muscle mass, boosting your metabolism and increasing your body's calorie-burning capacity.

Moreover, Pilates promotes mindfulness and body awareness, which can improve your relationship with food and support healthier eating habits. It's also a stress-reducing activity, which is essential as high stress levels can lead to weight gain.

However, it's crucial to view Pilates not as a quick fix for weight loss but as part of a balanced, sustainable lifestyle. It's a practice that nurtures your body, enhances your health, and supports your overall well-being, regardless of the number on the scale.

In conclusion, the world of Wall Pilates is layered with complexities and common misconceptions. It's our responsibility to separate the myths from the facts and understand this beautiful practice's true essence. As we continue to explore Wall Pilates, let's remember to keep an open mind, question the misconceptions, and celebrate the diversity and inclusivity this practice promotes. In the next chapter, we'll delve into the nitty-gritty of setting up your home studio – a crucial step towards starting your Wall Pilates practice. So, let's continue our adventure, one myth and one truth at a time.

Chapter 5: Your Personal Pilates Studio: Setting Up for Success

Imagine the thrill of embarking on a road trip. Your route is mapped out, your playlist ready, and your snacks packed. But before you hit the road, one vital step is ensuring your vehicle is in top shape. Just as your car is the foundation of your road trip, the wall is the cornerstone of your Wall Pilates practice. So, before we hit the road to fitness, let's ensure our 'vehicle' - our wall - is ready for the journey.

Wall Pilates, with its simplicity and versatility, is designed to fit seamlessly into your life. One of the most appealing aspects of this practice is that it can be done right in the comfort of your own home. All you need is a wall - no fancy gym membership or expensive equipment is required. But not just any wall will do. Let's explore how to find the perfect wall for your Wall Pilates practice.

Identifying Suitable Walls in Your Home

The first step in setting up your home Pilates studio is identifying a suitable wall. You might be thinking, "A wall is a wall, right?" But for Wall Pilates, there are a few key factors to consider.

First, look for a flat and even wall without any fixtures or obstructions. This will ensure you have enough space to perform a variety of exercises without any interruptions. An ideal wall is roughly the length of your body, allowing you to stretch out fully during specific exercises.

Next, consider the location of the wall. Is it in a quiet, well-lit area of your home? Is there enough space around it for you to move freely? Is it close to where you'd typically work out? Remember, convenience is key. The easier it is to access your workout space, the more likely you are to stick to your routine.

Assessing Wall Stability and Safety

Once you've identified a potential wall, the next step is to assess its stability. Remember, the wall will support some of your weight during your workouts, so it must be sturdy and solid. A thin or fragile wall may not provide the support you need and could lead to injuries.

So, how do you assess a wall's stability? A simple test is to press against the wall with your hands. If the wall feels firm and doesn't budge, it's likely sturdy enough for your workouts.

Safety is paramount in Wall Pilates. Ensure the wall's surface isn't slippery or rough, as this could cause accidents or discomfort during your workouts. Make sure the paint isn't chipping or peeling if the wall is painted.

Preparing the Wall for Pilates Exercises

Now that you've chosen your wall, it's time to prep it for your Wall Pilates sessions. This doesn't involve any drastic changes, just a few simple steps to ensure your wall is workout-ready.

First, make sure the wall is clean. Wipe it down with a damp cloth to remove any dust or dirt. This not only keeps your workout space hygienic but also prevents any dust particles from irritating your skin or eyes during your workout.

Next, if your wall is rough, consider smoothing it out. Sandpaper can help remove any minor rough patches. However, if the wall is very rough or uneven, choosing a different wall for your workouts might be best.

Finally, keep a small towel handy. You can use this to wipe down the wall after your workouts, keeping it clean and fresh for your next session.

The process of finding the perfect wall for your Wall Pilates practice might seem a bit meticulous, but remember, this wall is going to be your support system, your anchor, and your workout partner. So, take the time to choose wisely, assess thoroughly, and prepare carefully. A well-chosen wall enhances the safety and effectiveness of your workouts and contributes to a more enjoyable and fulfilling Wall Pilates experience.

Now, let's pause here. Take a moment to reflect on your chosen wall. Stand against it, feel its steadiness, its solidity. This wall is more than just a part of your home; it's about to become a part of your fitness journey, supporting you as you explore the wonderful world of Wall Pilates. So, here's to your wall - your partner in fitness, your companion in health, and your pathway to a stronger, more flexible, and more balanced you.

Essential Equipment for Wall Pilates

What makes Wall Pilates uniquely appealing is its simplicity - the fact that you can perform a full-body workout with minimal equipment. The star of your setup, of course, is the wall itself. But there are a few more pieces that can elevate your practice:

1. Yoga Mat: A good mat is a must-have for your wall Pilates sessions. It provides cushioning for your body and ensures a non-slip surface for your workouts. Opt for a mat that is thick enough to offer comfort yet firm enough to provide stability.

2. Yoga Blocks: These handy props can help modify certain exercises, making them more accessible. They can also be used to increase the intensity of some exercises, adding an extra challenge to your sessions.

3. Resistance Bands: These versatile tools can add a new dimension to your wall Pilates workouts. They provide resistance, helping to strengthen and tone your muscles.

4. Pilates Ball: This small, inflatable ball can be used for a variety of exercises. It can help deepen stretches, enhance stability, and target specific muscle groups.

5. Water Bottle: Staying hydrated, including wall Pilates, is crucial during any workout. Keep a water bottle nearby to quench your thirst throughout your session.

Remember, these are merely suggestions. Your wall Pilates setup should cater to your specific needs, preferences, and goals. Start with the basics and gradually add on as you progress in your practice.

Proper Placement and Installation of Equipment

Now that you've gathered your equipment, the next step is to arrange it in a functional and convenient way. Here are some tips to help you:

1. Yoga Mat: Position your mat perpendicular to the wall. This will provide ample space for a range of exercises, from standing moves to floor-based routines.

2. Yoga Blocks and Pilates Ball: These small props can be kept within reach, either at one end of your mat or on a nearby shelf. This ensures they are easily accessible whenever you need them.

3. Resistance Bands: If you use resistance bands, ensure they are safely secured. Some exercises may require you to loop the band around a sturdy object. In such cases, ensure the band is tightly fastened to prevent it from slipping during your workout.

4. Water Bottle: Keep your water bottle close by, ideally at the head of your mat. This way, you can stay hydrated without interrupting your flow.

Remember, the goal is to create a practical, clutter-free space conducive to focused workouts. So, take the time to arrange your equipment to best support your practice.

Maintaining and Caring for Your Equipment

Your wall Pilates equipment is an investment in your health and wellness. Like any investment, it requires care and maintenance to ensure its longevity. Here are some tips to keep your equipment in top shape:

1. Yoga Mat: Clean your mat after each workout. A simple wipe-down with a damp cloth and mild soap should do the trick. Allow your mat to air dry completely before rolling it up for storage.

2. Yoga Blocks and Pilates Ball: These props can be cleaned with a damp cloth and mild soap. Avoid using harsh chemicals, as they can damage the material.

3. Resistance Bands: Regularly inspect your bands for signs of wear and tear. If you notice any cracks or thinning, it's time to replace the band. To clean your bands, use a damp cloth and mild soap. Dry them thoroughly before storing them to prevent damage.

4. Water Bottle: Clean your water bottle after every workout to prevent bacteria build-up. Most water bottles are dishwasher safe, but always check the manufacturer's instructions to be sure.

Maintaining your equipment extends its lifespan and ensures a safe and hygienic workout environment. It's a small step that can make a big difference in your wall Pilates experience.

So, there you have it - your personal Pilates studio right in your own home! But remember, this setup is not set in stone. Feel free to tweak and adjust as you progress in your practice. After all, your wall Pilates space should reflect your unique fitness journey, growing and evolving just as you do.

Creating a Calm and Motivating Atmosphere. Choosing the Right Lighting

The quality of light in your Wall Pilates space can greatly impact your workout experience. Ideally, you want a natural and artificial light blend to create a warm, inviting atmosphere. If your chosen wall is near a window, take advantage of the daylight for your morning or afternoon sessions. The natural light will energize you and enhance your mood as you exercise.

You'll need some artificial lighting for evening workouts or on cloudy days. Opt for soft, white light that mimics natural daylight. Avoid harsh, direct lights that can strain your eyes. A floor lamp with an adjustable brightness setting could be a good choice, allowing you to control the intensity of the light as per your preference.

Experiment with different lighting options and observe how they affect your mood and energy levels during your workout. The goal is to create a light setting that keeps you alert yet relaxed throughout your session.

Selecting Motivational Decor

The decor of your Wall Pilates space can serve as a source of inspiration and motivation. Start by choosing a color palette that resonates with you. Soft, earthy tones create a calming environment, while brighter hues energize you.

Next, consider adding some motivational elements to your space. This could be a framed quote that inspires you, a vision board with images of your fitness goals, or a progress chart where you can track your achievements.

However, remember to keep the decor minimal and functional. Too many elements can be distracting and may obstruct your movements. The focus should be on creating a space that motivates you and enhances your Wall Pilates experience.

Incorporating Elements of Nature

Bringing nature into your workout space can have numerous benefits. Plants, for instance, add a touch of green and improve air quality. Choose low-maintenance indoor plants that thrive in your home's light conditions.

You can also incorporate other natural elements like a small water fountain or a bowl of pebbles. The sound of trickling water can be very soothing and enhance the meditative aspect of your Wall Pilates practice.

Another idea is to use aromatherapy to create a refreshing and calming atmosphere. Essential oils like lavender or eucalyptus can be diffused during your workout to invigorate your senses and deepen your relaxation.

Remember, your Wall Pilates space is an extension of your personality and your fitness journey. It should be a place where you feel comfortable, motivated, and inspired. So, take some time to create a space that truly reflects you and supports your Wall Pilates practice. It's not just about setting up a physical space; it's about creating an environment that nurtures your body, calms your mind, and lifts your spirit. So, go ahead and create a space where you can truly enjoy your Wall Pilates experience.

Correct Posture and Alignment: A Pillar of Wall Pilates

Before we get moving with our wall workouts, let's first lay down some safety guidelines. The first and perhaps most important is understanding the role of posture and alignment in Pilates.

Imagine your body as a well-oiled machine. Each part needs to be in its right place for the machine to function optimally. In Pilates, this is where posture and alignment come into play. They ensure that your body parts are positioned correctly, thus optimizing your workout and minimizing the risk of injuries.

In Wall Pilates, alignment starts with your back against the wall. Your head, shoulders, and hips should touch the wall, and there should be a small space in the lower back area. This neutral spine position serves as the starting point for most wall Pilates exercises.

As you move through various exercises, always be mindful of your alignment. Always keep your neck long, shoulders down and relaxed, and hips level. This alignment awareness not only improves the effectiveness of your workouts but also helps prevent strain and injury.

Warm-Up and Cool-Down Routines: The Alpha and Omega of Your Workouts

Now that we've sorted our posture and alignment let's move on to the next safety guideline - the importance of warm-up and cool-down routines.

Think of your body as a car engine. You wouldn't slam on the accelerator without warming it up first. Similarly, before you start your Wall Pilates exercises, preparing your body with a good warm-up routine is important. This could be as simple as marching in place, doing some shoulder rolls, or performing a few gentle stretches. The aim is to gradually increase your heart rate, warm up your muscles, and prime your body for the workout ahead.

At the other end of your workout is the cool-down phase. Just as you wouldn't abruptly stop a car at full speed, you shouldn't abruptly stop your workout, either. A cool-down routine allows your heart rate and breathing to return to normal gradually. It also helps prevent muscle stiffness and soreness. A few minutes of slow, gentle stretching can serve as an effective cool-down routine.

Remember, every good workout has a beginning and an end. The warm-up is your beginning; the cool-down is your end. They are the alpha and omega of your workout and should never be skipped.

Injury Prevention and First Aid: Being Prepared for the Unexpected

Even with good posture, alignment, and proper warm-up and cool-down routines, accidents can still happen. That's why it's essential to be prepared for unexpected injuries.

Prevention is the first step. Always keep your workout space clear of clutter to avoid tripping or slipping. Use a good-quality mat that provides enough cushioning and grip. Listen to your body, and do not push yourself beyond your limits. If an exercise causes pain or discomfort, stop immediately and modify as needed. Despite these precautions, injuries can still occur. In such cases, it's important to know some basic first aid. Remember the RICE protocol - Rest, Ice, Compression, and Elevation for minor injuries like sprains or strains.

For more serious injuries, seek professional medical help immediately. Keep your doctor's number handy and let your family members know when you are working out, especially if you are alone at home.

Safety should always be your top priority in Wall Pilates. With these guidelines in place, you can ensure that your practice is effective, enjoyable, and safe.

So, there you have it - your Wall Pilates studio in your home. From finding the perfect wall to setting up your equipment, creating a motivating atmosphere, and ensuring safety, you are ready to embark on your Wall Pilates adventure. As you stand against your wall, feel its steadiness, its support. This wall is not just a part of your home; it's about to become a part of your fitness story, a story of strength, flexibility, and holistic wellness. So, take a deep breath, brace yourself, and let's get moving! On to the next chapter, where the real fun begins - your first Wall Pilates moves.

Chapter 6: Your Own Pilates Wall: A Gateway to Transformation

Picture this: you're standing in front of a blank canvas, brush in hand, palette full of vibrant colors, ready to create your masterpiece. The canvas is your opportunity, your potential. This is the same feeling you should have when you stand in front of your wall, ready to start your Wall Pilates practice. Your wall is your canvas, and you're about to create a masterpiece of strength, flexibility, and wellness.

This chapter marks an exciting milestone in your Wall Pilates journey. It's time to get up close and personal with your wall. We'll learn how to choose the right wall, prepare it for your workouts, and ensure your practice is safe and effective. Let's dive in and get comfortable with the wall!

Visual Guide to Wall Pilates Positions. Decoding Position Diagrams

To get the most out of your Wall Pilates practice, it's important to understand how to interpret position diagrams. These diagrams are visual representations of various Wall Pilates positions and are designed to guide you in correctly performing each exercise.

This visual cue gives you a clear picture of what the final position should look like. However, it's crucial to remember that these diagrams are a guide, not an absolute rule. Everyone's body is different, and what works for one person may not work for another. Therefore, always listen to your body and adjust the positions as necessary.

Pictorial Walkthrough of Positions

Let's take a pictorial walkthrough of some commonly used Wall Pilates positions to assist your understanding further.

-
-
-

- **Wall Stand:** Stand with your back against the wall. Your feet should be hip-width apart, and about a foot away from the wall. The back of your head, shoulders, and hips should be touching the wall. This is your starting position for many Wall Pilates exercises.

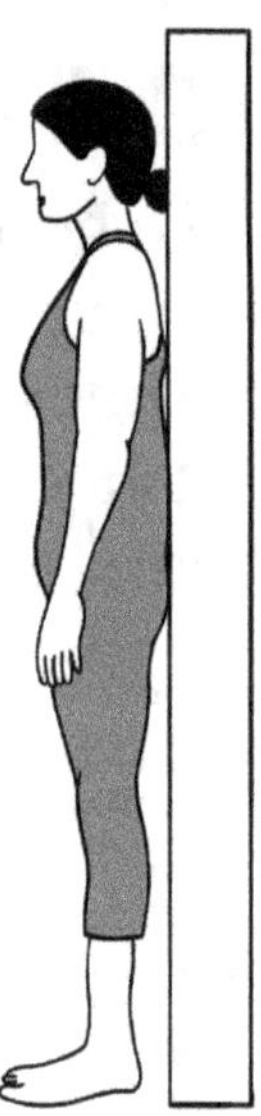

- **Wall Slide:** From the Wall Stand position, bend your knees and slide down the wall until your knees are bent at a 90-degree angle. Make sure your knees are directly above your ankles. This position works your lower body and core.

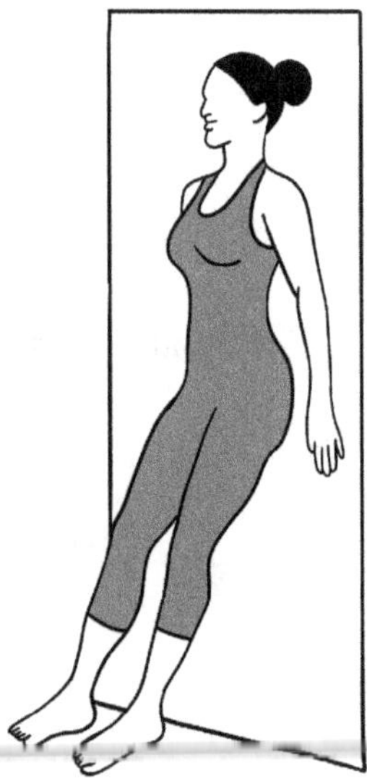 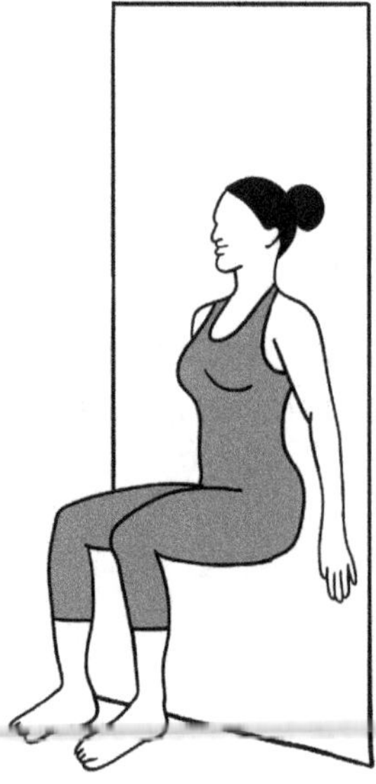

- **Wall Push-up:** Stand facing the wall, arms-length away. Place your hands on the wall slightly wider than shoulder-width apart. Bend your elbows and bring your chest towards the wall, keeping your body straight. Push back to the starting position. This position targets your upper body.

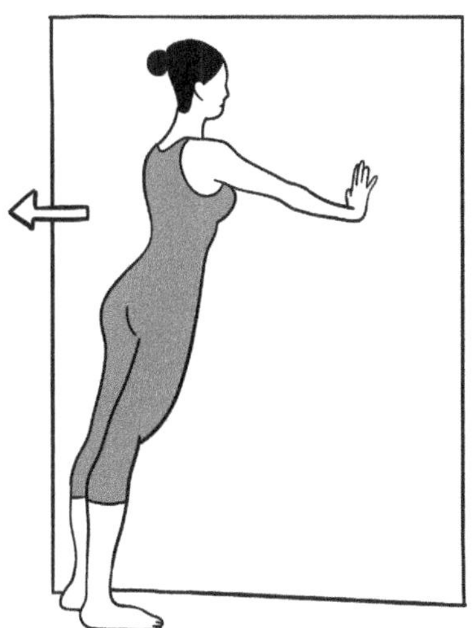 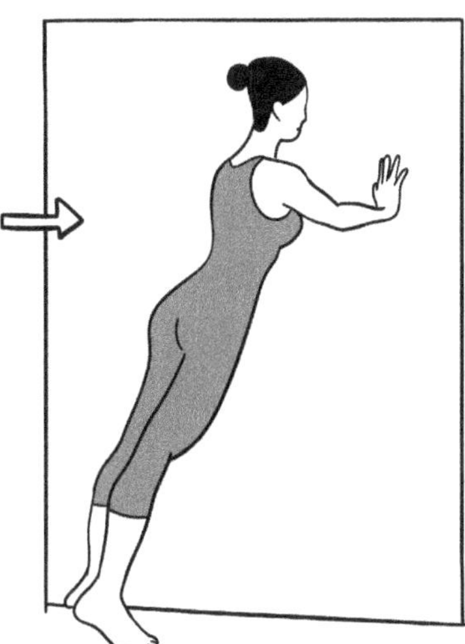

- **Wall Plank:** Stand facing the wall. Walk your feet back and lean forward until your body is at an angle to the wall. Your hands should be on the wall, shoulder-width apart, and your body should form a straight line from your head to your heels. This position is a full-body workout with an emphasis on the core.

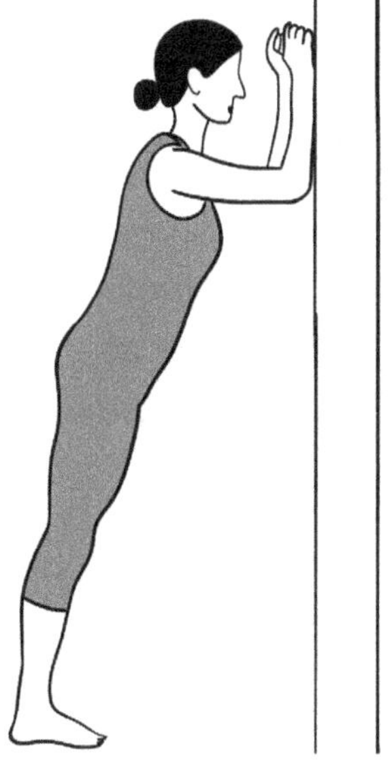

- **Wall Bridge:** Lie on your back with your feet on the wall, knees bent at a 90-degree angle. Lift your hips off the floor, pressing your feet into the wall. This position targets your glutes, hamstrings, and lower back.

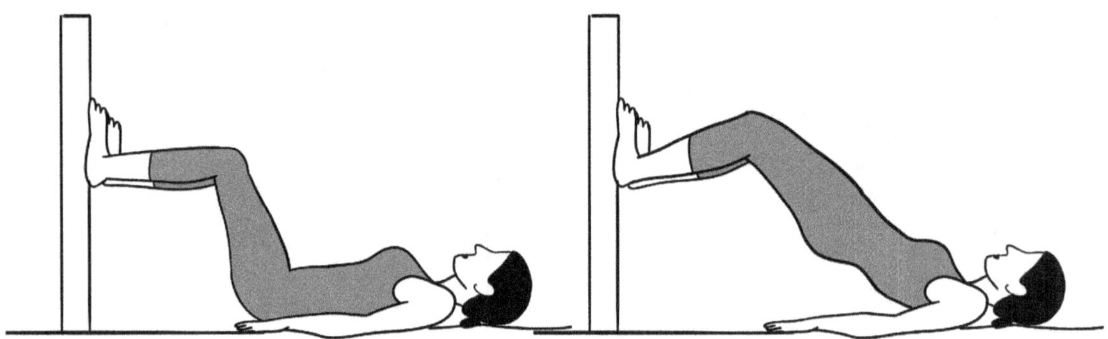

By familiarizing yourself with these diagrams, you'll be able to set up each position correctly and get the maximum benefit from your Wall Pilates workouts.

Advanced Techniques

As you progress in your Wall Pilates practice, you might come across diagrams for more advanced positions. These positions typically involve more complex movements or greater strength and flexibility. Examples could include the Wall Handstand, Wall Pike, or Wall Mountain Climbers.

When attempting these advanced positions, it's essential to maintain proper form and alignment. It's also crucial to listen to your body and only attempt these positions when you feel ready. If you're unsure, it's always a good idea to consult a certified Pilates instructor or a fitness professional.

Remember, the goal of Wall Pilates is not to achieve the most advanced positions. It's about improving your strength, flexibility, and overall fitness. It's about enjoying the process, celebrating your progress, and feeling good in your body. So, take your time, be patient with yourself, and most importantly, have fun with your practice!

Your First Wall Pilates Moves

Wall Roll Down: A Gentle Start

Let's start your Wall Pilates journey with a gentle yet effective exercise: the Wall Roll Down. This exercise targets your entire body, with an emphasis on your core and spine.

To perform the Wall Roll Down, start in **Wall Stand** position. Inhale deeply, and as you exhale, tuck your chin towards your chest and slowly roll down, one vertebra at a time. Allow your arms to hang loosely as you roll down as far as you can go comfortably. Inhale at the bottom, then exhale and slowly roll back up to the starting position.

The **Wall Roll Down** is a great exercise to start your workout as it warms up your muscles, mobilizes your spine, and helps you tune into your body.

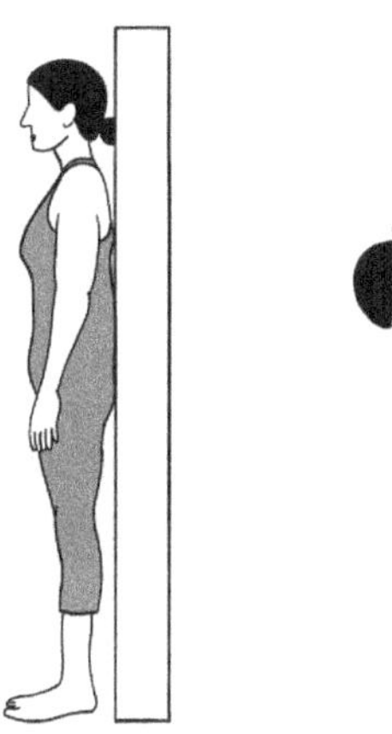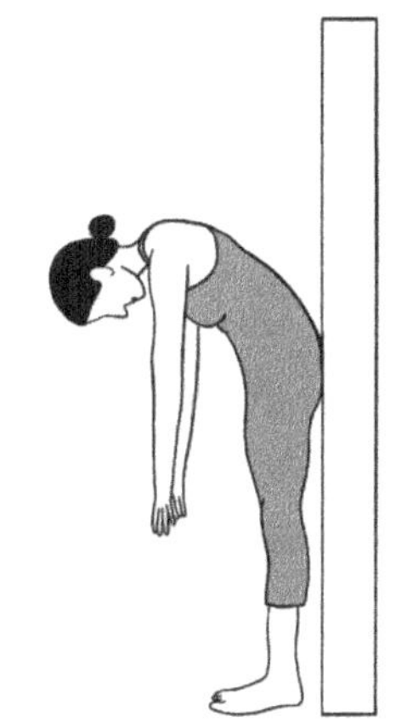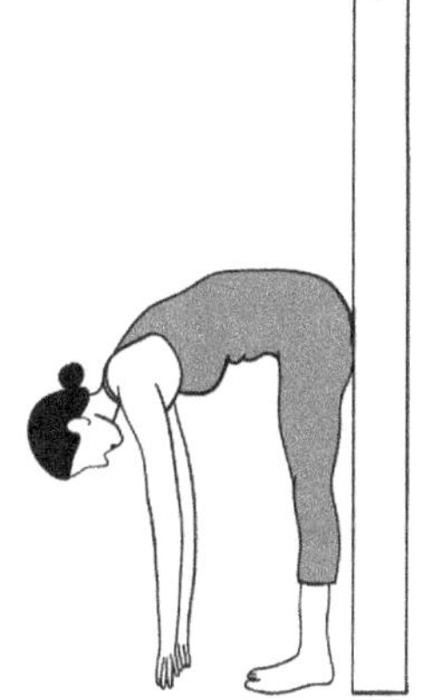

Wall Push-Up: Strength in Simplicity

Next, let's move on to the Wall Push-Up, a simple exercise that packs a punch. The Wall Push-Up targets your upper body, particularly your arms, shoulders, and chest, while also engaging your core. To do the Wall Push-Up, start by standing facing the wall, arms-length away. Place your hands on the wall, slightly wider than shoulder-width apart. Bend your elbows and bring your chest towards the wall, keeping your body straight. Push back to the starting position.

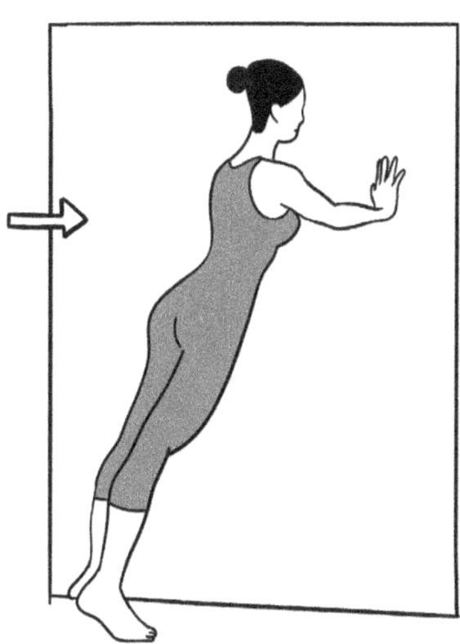

Remember to keep your core engaged throughout the exercise. The Wall Push-Up can be modified to suit different fitness levels by adjusting the distance between you and the wall.

Wall Squat: Lower Body Power

Lastly, let's tackle the Wall Squat, an exercise that targets your lower body, particularly your thighs and glutes. The Wall Squat also engages your core and improves your balance and stability.

From Wall Stand position, walk your feet about a foot away from the wall. Inhale, and as you exhale, slide down the wall, bending your knees until they are at a 90-degree angle. Make sure your knees are directly above your ankles. Hold this position for a few seconds, then slide back up the wall to the starting position.

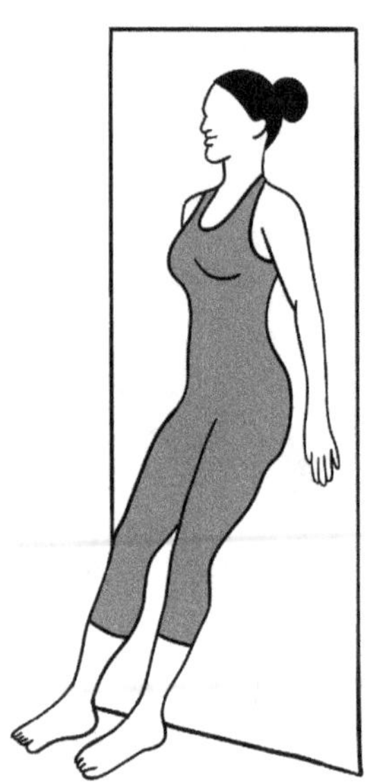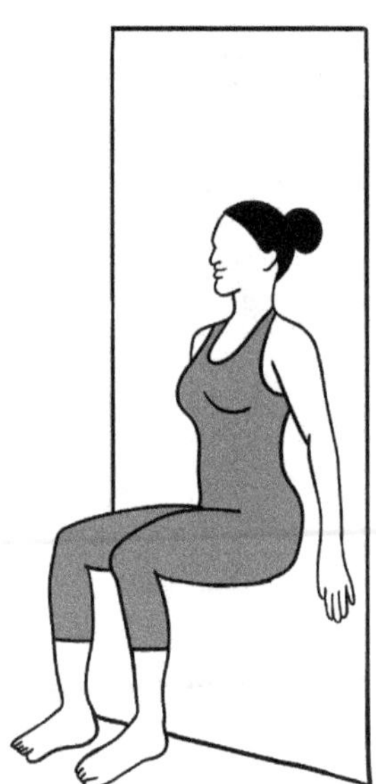

The Wall Squat is a versatile exercise that can be modified or progressed to match your fitness level. For example, you can hold the squat position for a longer time or add a resistance band around your thighs to increase the challenge.

Remember, these are just your first steps in Wall Pilates. There's a whole world of exercises and variations to explore as you progress in your practice. So, take it one step at a time, enjoy the journey, and look forward to all the exciting challenges and achievements ahead.

Correct Alignment and Posture: The Cornerstone of Effective Practice

Understanding Neutral Spine: The Foundation of Alignment

In Wall Pilates, correct alignment starts with understanding the concept of a neutral spine. A neutral spine means maintaining the natural curves of your spine - a slight inward curve at your lower back, a slight outward curve at your upper back, and a slight inward curve at your neck. This position allows for optimal balance and force distribution in your body.

Aim to maintain a neutral spine when standing against the wall for your Wall Pilates workout. The back of your head, upper back, and hips should be touching the wall, and there should be a small space in the lower back area. Imagine you're holding a small grape in the curve of your lower back - it shouldn't be squished, but it shouldn't fall off, either.

Importance of Pelvic Alignment: Balancing Your Foundation

Your pelvis is the foundation of your alignment in Wall Pilates. When your pelvis is in the correct position, it's easier to maintain a neutral spine and move effectively.

In Wall Pilates, aim for a neutral pelvis position. This means your pelvis should not be tilting excessively forward or backwards. A good way to find your neutral pelvis is to place your hands on your hip bones and imagine them as a car's headlights. The headlights should be shining straight ahead, not up towards the ceiling or down towards the floor.

Remember, achieving a neutral spine and pelvis might initially feel a little unfamiliar, especially if you're used to poor postural habits. But with practice and awareness, it will become more natural and comfortable.

Head and Neck Positioning: Aligning the Top of the Chain

Lastly, let's talk about the alignment of your head and neck - the top of your alignment chain. In Wall Pilates, your head and neck should be in a neutral position, in line with your spine.

A common mistake is to jut the chin forward or tuck it too much into the chest. To avoid this, imagine a string attached to the crown of your head, pulling you up towards the ceiling. This will help lengthen your neck and align your head correctly.

Remember, proper alignment is a dynamic process, not a static state. It's about maintaining balance and control as you move through different positions and exercises. Always be mindful of your alignment, and don't hesitate to adjust as needed.

Building Strength and Flexibility: The Dual Goals of Wall Pilates

Wall Leg Slides: A Slide to Strength and Stability

One of the key benefits of Wall Pilates is its ability to build strength, particularly core strength. A great exercise to achieve this is the Wall Leg Slides. This exercise targets your core while also working your lower body.

To perform Wall Leg Slides, start by lying on your back with your hips close to the wall, knees bent, and feet flat on the wall. Slowly straighten one leg, sliding your heel up the wall, then slide it back down. Repeat with the other leg.

Remember to engage your core and maintain a neutral spine throughout the exercise. The Wall Leg Slides can be modified by adjusting the distance between your hips and the wall.

Wall Angels: Stretch and Strengthen

Wall Angels are another excellent exercise that combines strength and flexibility. This exercise targets your upper body, particularly your shoulders and back.

To do Wall Angels, stand with your back against the wall, feet about a foot away from the wall. Bend your elbows and press your arms against the wall in a "W" shape. Slide your arms up the wall, straightening them as much as you can while keeping them in contact with the wall, then slide them back down to the "W" position.

Wall Angels strengthen your upper body, improve your posture, and increase your shoulder flexibility. They can be modified by adjusting your distance from the wall or using a resistance band.

Wall Plank: A Full-Body Challenge

Let's end this section with a full-body exercise - the Wall Plank. This exercise engages almost all your major muscle groups, particularly emphasising your core.

To perform the Wall Plank, stand facing the wall. Walk your feet back and lean forward until your body is at an angle to the wall. Your hands should be on the wall, shoulder-width apart, and your body should form a straight line from your head to your heels. Hold this position for a few seconds, then return to the starting position.

The Wall Plank is a versatile exercise that can be modified or progressed to match your fitness level. You can adjust the angle of your body to make the exercise easier or harder or add variations like a leg lift or knee tuck for an extra challenge.

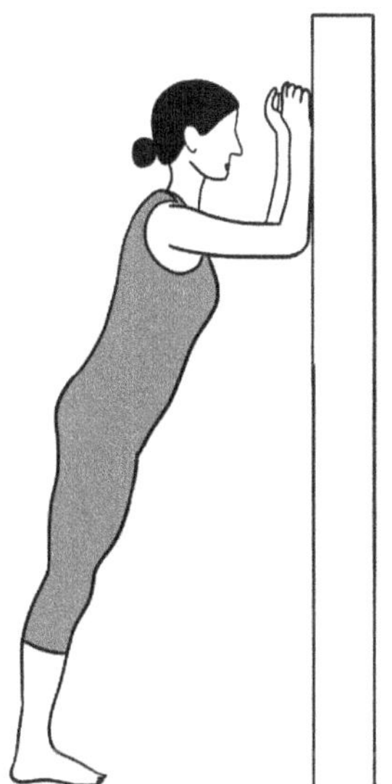 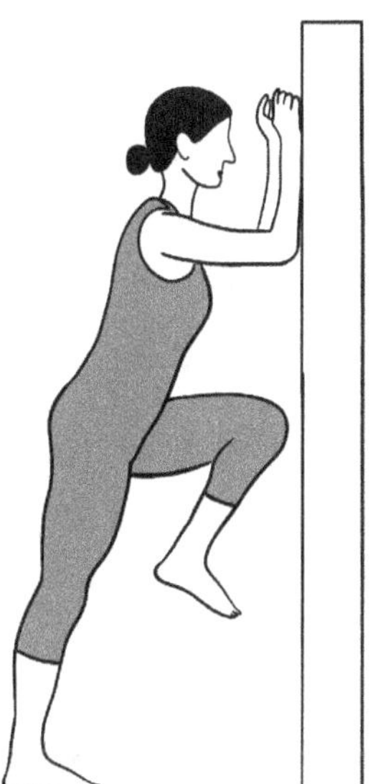

Remember, Wall Pilates is not about doing the hardest exercises or the most repetitions. It's about improving your strength, flexibility, and overall fitness at your own pace. It's about enjoying the process, celebrating your progress, and feeling good in your body. So, take it one step at a time, enjoy the journey, and look forward to all the exciting challenges and achievements ahead.

As you explore these exercises and feel comfortable with your wall, remind yourself why you started this journey. Remember the vision you had for your health, your body, and your well-being. With each Wall Roll Down, each Wall Push-Up, and each Wall Squat, you're getting closer to that vision. You're not just working out; you're creating a masterpiece of strength, flexibility, and wellness. And the best part? This is just the beginning. There's a whole world of Wall

Pilates to explore and endless possibilities to discover. So, keep practicing, keep exploring, and keep creating your masterpiece. Your Wall Pilates adventure is only just getting started.

Empowering Your Body: Cultivating Strength and Flexibility

Wall Leg Slides: Elevating Your Fitness Quotient

Now let's immerse ourselves in an exercise that's as invigorating as it is foundational - the Wall Leg Slides. It's simple, effective, and perfect for beginners and seasoned practitioners alike. This exercise is your stepping stone to a stronger core and more stable lower body.

To perform Wall Leg Slides, begin by lying on your back with your feet resting on the wall. Your knees should be bent at a comfortable 90-degree angle. Now comes the exciting part. As you exhale, slowly straighten one leg, sliding your heel up the wall. Feel the stretch in your hamstring and the engagement in your core. As you inhale, slide your heel back down, returning to the starting position. Repeat with the other leg.

The Wall Leg Slides are not just about moving your legs. It's about moving with control, activating your core, and cultivating a deeper mind-body connection. So go ahead, slide into your strength and stability with this versatile exercise.

Wall Angels: Nurturing Mobility and Strength

Next on our list is an exercise that's as heavenly as it sounds - the Wall Angels. It's a fantastic way to open up your chest, strengthen your back, and improve your posture.

Begin by standing with your back against the wall, feet hip-width apart. Bend your elbows and press your arms against the wall in a "W" shape. Now, imagine you're creating snow angels on the wall. As you inhale, slide your arms up the wall, straightening them as much as you can while keeping them in contact with the wall. As you exhale, slide them back down to the "W" position.

Feel the stretch in your chest, the strength in your back, and the rhythm of your breath. The Wall Angels is a celebration of your body's mobility and strength. So, spread your wings and soar high with this invigorating exercise.

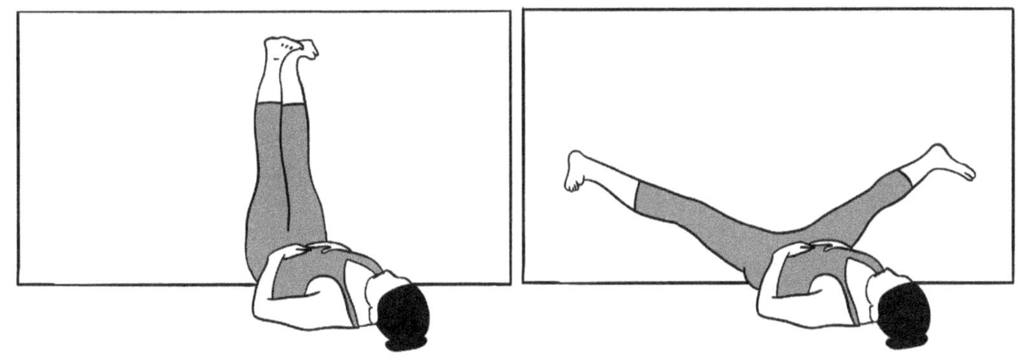

Wall Split

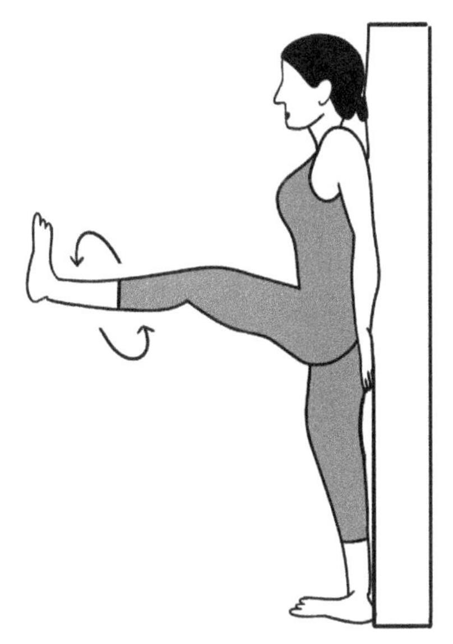

Leg Circle

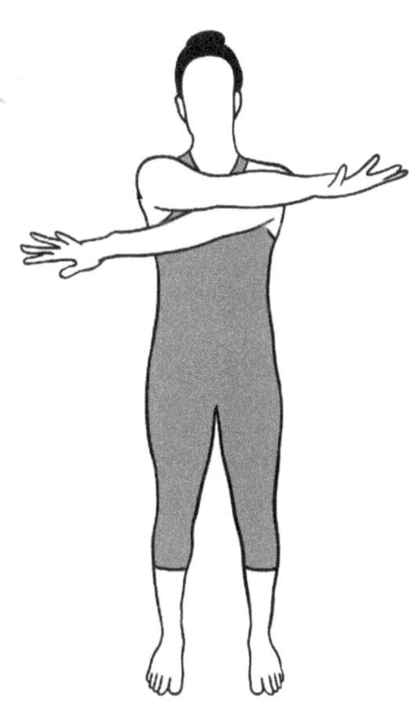

Wall Scissors

Make a Difference with Your Review

Review Request:" **Wall Pilates for Women: 28-Day Challenge from Beginner to Advanced**

How to Share Your Thoughts:
- Visit the Book's Page: Go to the book's page on your preferred platform (Amazon, Goodreads, etc.).
- Compose Your Review: Share what you loved about the book covered.
- Rate the Book: Give it a star rating that reflects your overall impression.

Bonus: The Power of Generosity
As a token of our appreciation, we invite you to consider the power of generosity. Your review helps fellow readers and supports an author who has poured time and expertise into creating this book. Thank you for considering our request. Your generosity in sharing your thoughts can make a world of difference.

With thanks,

Grace Hartley

Skilset Publishing

Chapter 7: Your Journey Begins: Embracing the 28-Day Wall Pilates Program

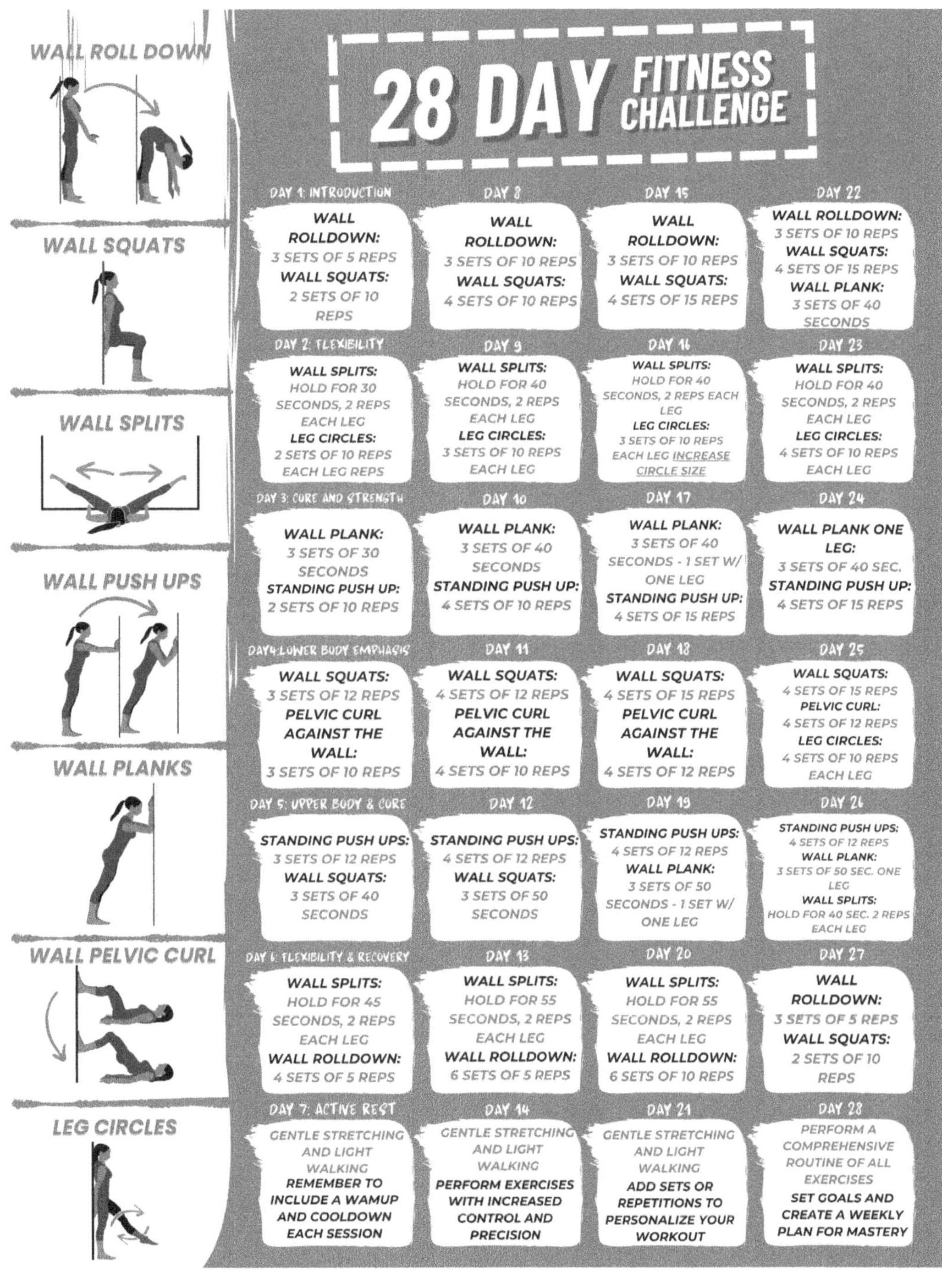

5-Minute Pilates Warm-Up Routine

This warm-up routine is designed to gently activate various muscle groups and increase blood flow, preparing your body for wall Pilates. Remember to do these exercises at a comfortable pace and intensity to avoid overexertion before your main workout.

- **March in Place** (1 minute): Start by standing with your feet hip-width apart. Begin marching in place, lifting your knees and gently swinging your arms. This helps to increase your heart rate and warm up your muscles.

- **Shoulder Rolls** (1 minute): While standing, roll your shoulders in a circular motion, first forwards for 30 seconds and then backwards for another 30 seconds. This helps to loosen up the shoulder and neck area.

- **Side Stretches** (1 minute): Stand with your feet slightly wider than hip-width apart. Raise one arm overhead and lean to the opposite side, stretching the side of your body. Hold for a few seconds, then switch to the other side. Alternate sides for the full minute.

- **Gentle Squats** (1 minute): Stand with your feet hip-width apart. Bend your knees and lower your hips as if you are going to sit in a chair, then rise back up. Keep the squats shallow and focus on warming up the legs and glutes.

- **Ankle Rolls** (1 minute): Lift one foot off the ground and roll your ankle in a circular motion. Do this for 30 seconds, then switch to the other foot. This helps to warm up the ankles, improving mobility and reducing the risk of injury.

- ### 5-Minute Pilates Cool-Down Routine

Remember to perform these exercises in a controlled manner, paying attention to your body's limits. This routine should help you safely prepare for and recover from your 20-minute wall Pilates program.

- **Wall Stretch (**1 minute): Stand facing the wall, place your hands on the wall at shoulder height, and step back a few feet. Lean forward, keeping your heels on the ground and feeling a stretch in your shoulders and hamstrings.

- **Calf Stretch (**1 minute): Facing the wall, step one foot back, keeping it flat on the ground. Bend your front knee, keeping your back leg straight. Hold for 30 seconds and switch legs.

- **Spinal Twist** (1 minute): Sit on the ground with your legs extended. Cross one leg over the other, placing the foot flat on the ground. Twist your torso toward the bent knee, using your arm for leverage against the knee. Hold for 30 seconds and switch sides.

- **Hamstring Stretch** (1 minute): Sit with your back against the wall, legs extended in front of you. Reach forward toward your toes, feeling the stretch in your hamstrings and lower back. Hold the stretch.

- **Deep Breathing** (1 minute): Conclude with deep breathing as you did in the warm-up. Sit comfortably with your back straight, inhale deeply through your nose, and exhale slowly through your mouth. Focus on relaxing your entire body.

Picture this: you're standing at the base of a mountain, eyes fixed on the peak, heart filled with a mix of excitement and anticipation. You're about to climb this mountain, one step at a time, one day at a time. Now, swap the mountain with our 28-Day Wall Pilates program. Yes, it's going to be a climb. But every climb begins with a single step, and that first step is setting your goals.

In the realm of fitness, goals are your guiding stars. They give your efforts a direction, your journey a purpose. They are the 'why' behind your 'what' and 'how'. In this section, we'll explore how to set effective, achievable fitness goals and how these goals can empower your Wall Pilates practice.

Setting Your Goals for the Program

Defining Personal Fitness Goals

What does fitness mean to you? Is it about losing a few pounds, toning your body, improving your posture, or enhancing your overall well-being? It could be all of these or none of these. It could be something uniquely personal to you. The first step in setting your goals is defining what fitness means to you.

Take a quiet moment for yourself. Sit comfortably, close your eyes, and visualize your ideal state of fitness. What do you see? What do you feel? What do you wish to achieve through your Wall Pilates practice? Write these down in as much detail as you can. This is your fitness vision.

Importance of SMART Goals

Now that you have your fitness vision, it's time to translate it into SMART goals. SMART stands for Specific, Measurable, Achievable, Relevant, and Time-bound. Let's break it down:

- **Specific:** Instead of "I want to get fit," try "I want to be able to perform a full Wall Plank for one minute."

- **Measurable:** Make sure you can track your progress. Instead of "I want to feel stronger," try "I want to increase the number of Wall Push-ups I can do."

- **Achievable**: Set goals that challenge you but are still within your reach. It's better to start with smaller goals and gradually increase the challenge.

- **Relevant:** Your goals should align with your fitness vision and your personal values.

- **Time-bound:** Give your goals a timeframe. When do you want to achieve this goal? Setting a time limit creates a sense of urgency and can motivate you to take action.

Visualization Techniques

With your SMART goals in hand, it's time to bring in a powerful tool - visualization. Visualization involves creating a mental image of achieving your goals. It activates your creative subconscious, generates positive emotions, and programs your brain to recognize the resources you need to achieve your goals.

Find a quiet, comfortable space where you won't be disturbed. Close your eyes and take a few deep breaths. Now, imagine yourself achieving your fitness goals. If your goal is to do a full Wall Plank for one minute, visualize yourself doing just that. Feel the strength in your core, hear your steady breath, and see the smile of accomplishment on your face. Make the image as clear and detailed as possible.

Visualization is not just daydreaming. It's a powerful technique used by successful people in all fields, from athletes to entrepreneurs. By visualizing your success, you're priming your mind to make it a reality.

So, there you have it - the first step in your 28-day Wall Pilates Program. By setting your fitness goals, you're not just planning your journey but also powering it. Your goals are now the roadmap to your success, motivation on the challenging days, and celebration on the victorious ones. So, cherish this moment. You've taken the first step on your Wall Pilates journey, and every step that follows will bring you closer to your goals, your vision, and your peak. Are you ready? Let's climb!

Week-by-Week Program Breakdown

Week 1: Foundation and Familiarization

Welcome to the first week of your Wall Pilates program, a week of discovery and understanding. This week is about acquainting yourself with Wall Pilates and setting a solid base for the weeks to come.

Start by exploring the basic Wall Pilates exercises introduced in the previous chapter. Pay attention to your form and alignment as you perform each exercise. Remember, it's not about how many repetitions you can do but how well you can do each one.

As you familiarize yourself with the exercises, also take note of how your body feels before, during, and after each workout. How does your body respond to different exercises? Which movements feel challenging, and which ones come naturally? These observations will help you better understand your body and tailor your Wall Pilates practice to suit your needs and goals.

Week 1 is also a time to cultivate consistency. Try to establish a regular workout schedule that fits seamlessly into your daily routine. Whether it's a morning session to jumpstart your day, an afternoon break to shake off the day's stress, or an evening workout to wind down before bed, find a time that works for you and stick to it.

Week 2: Building Strength and Stamina

As you step into week 2, you're ready to take your practice up a notch. This week is about building strength and stamina, pushing your boundaries, and challenging your limits.

Continue with the foundational exercises, but add a few more repetitions or hold each position for a bit longer. Remember to maintain correct form and alignment, even as you increase the intensity of your workouts.

Week 2 is also a time to start exploring modifications that can make each exercise more challenging. For instance, you could add a resistance band to your Wall Squat or perform the Wall Push-Up on your toes instead of flat feet. These little tweaks can significantly increase the challenge level of your workouts, helping you build strength and stamina.

Also, continue to be mindful of your body and how it feels. Are there certain exercises that you find particularly challenging? Are there areas of your body that feel stronger or more flexible? Use these insights to personalize your Wall Pilates practice further.

Week 3: Introducing Intermediate Moves

Week 3 marks the halfway point of your 28-Day Wall Pilates program, and it's time to introduce some intermediate moves. This week is about expanding your workout repertoire, exploring new challenges, and continuing to build on the strength and stamina you've developed in the past two weeks.

Start by adding a few intermediate exercises to your routine. These could include exercises like the Wall Plank with Knee Tuck or the Wall Bridge with Leg Lift. As always, pay attention to your form and alignment, and only progress to these exercises if you feel comfortable and ready.

Remember, each new exercise is a chance to learn and grow. Don't be discouraged if you find some moves challenging. Take it slow, listen to your body, and modify as needed. With time and practice, you'll be able to master these intermediate moves and reap their benefits.

Week 4: Advanced Techniques and Consolidation

As you enter the final week of your 28-Day Wall Pilates program, it's time to consolidate what you've learned and introduce some advanced techniques. This week is about refining your practice, pushing your limits, and celebrating how far you've come.

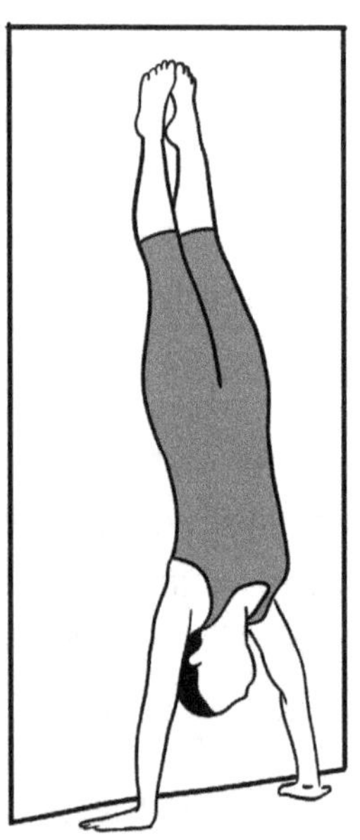

Continue with your regular workouts, but try to incorporate at least one advanced move into each session. This could be the Wall Handstand, the Wall Mountain Climbers, or any other advanced move that you feel ready to tackle. Remember, these moves should be challenging but not painful. Always listen to your body and only attempt advanced moves if you feel comfortable and ready.

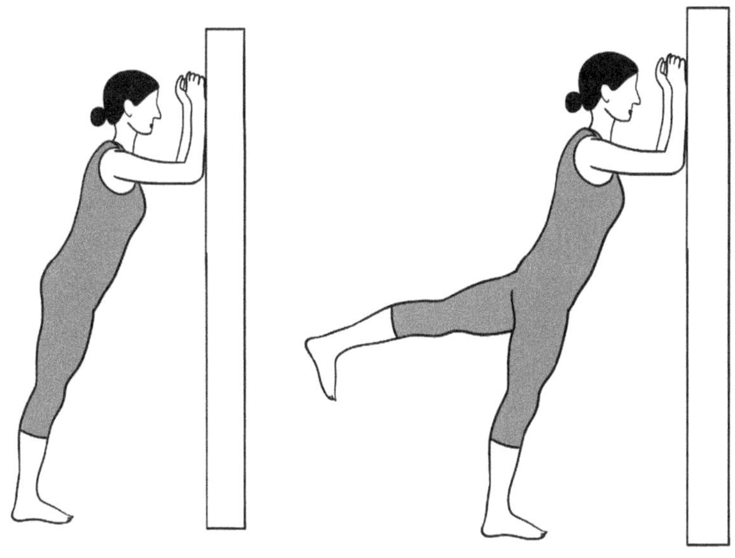

Arabesque

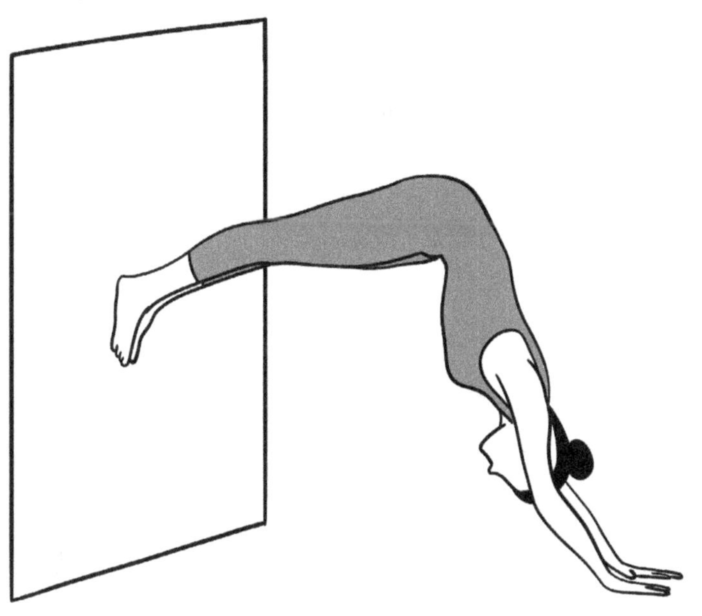

Wall Pike

Week 4 is also a time to reflect on your progress and celebrate your achievements. Look back at your fitness goals and see how far you've come. Celebrate each small victory, each hurdle overcome, each moment of strength, flexibility, and resilience. You've climbed the mountain, one step, one breath, one day at a time. And now, you're standing at the peak, basking in the glow of your achievement. But remember, this is not the end. It's just the beginning of many more Wall Pilates adventures to come.

Tracking Your Progress

Keeping a Workout Journal: Your Personal Fitness Diary

Think of a workout journal as your personal fitness diary, a space where you can record your exercises, reps, sets, and feelings during each workout. This simple habit can have a profound impact on your Wall Pilates practice.

Start by noting down the exercises you perform each day. Include specifics like the number of sets and reps, the intensity level, and any modifications you made. Also, jot down how you felt during and after each workout. Were some exercises challenging? Did you feel energized or exhausted after your session? These notes can provide valuable insights into your fitness levels and progress.

A workout journal also allows you to plan your future workouts. You can identify patterns, discover what works best for you, and plan your sessions accordingly. Plus, it's a great motivation booster. Looking back at your entries and seeing how far you've come can be incredibly motivating.

Measuring Physical Changes: Beyond the Scale

While relying on the scale to measure your progress is tempting, it's important to remember that physical changes involve much more than just weight loss. Wall Pilates helps you build lean muscle, improve posture, enhance flexibility, and boost overall fitness. These changes may not always reflect on the scale, but they significantly affect your health and well-being.

So, how can you measure these physical changes? Here are a few ideas:

- **Progress photos**: Take photos of yourself at the start of the program and then every week after that. You'll be able to see changes in your posture, muscle tone, and overall physique.

- **Body measurements:** Use a measuring tape to track changes in your body measurements. Areas to measure include your waist, hips, thighs, and arms.

- **Strength and endurance:** Keep track of how your strength and endurance improve over time. For example, are you able to hold a Wall Plank for longer? Can you do more Wall Push-ups than when you started?

- **Flexibility:** Notice improvements in your flexibility. Can you stretch further in your Wall Roll Down? Are your Wall Squats becoming smoother and more fluid?

Remember, everybody is unique, and changes happen at different rates. Be patient with yourself, and celebrate each improvement, no matter how small.

Assessing Mental and Emotional Growth: The Mind-Body Connection

Wall Pilates is not just a physical practice; it's also a mental and emotional journey. It helps you cultivate mindfulness, manage stress, and boost your mood. These mental and emotional changes are just as important as physical ones and deserve to be tracked and celebrated.

Here are a few ways to assess your mental and emotional growth:

- **Mindfulness:** Notice improvements in your mindfulness. Are you more aware of your body and its movements? Do you feel more present during your workouts?

- **Mood and energy levels:** Pay attention to your mood and energy levels. Do you feel more positive and energized after your Wall Pilates sessions?

- **Stress levels:** Assess your stress levels. Has your Wall Pilates practice helped you manage stress better?

- **Self-confidence:** Observe changes in your self-confidence. Do you feel more confident and comfortable in your body?

So, as you track your progress, don't forget to consider all aspects of your well-being. After all, the ultimate goal of your Wall Pilates practice is not just to transform your body but also to cultivate a balanced, healthy, and fulfilling lifestyle.

Charting Your Progress: A Visual Guide to Transformation

The Role of a Progress Chart in Your Wall Pilates Practice

The allure of Wall Pilates lies in its simplicity and effectiveness, but its true beauty unfolds when we witness our growth and transformation over time. This is where a progress chart comes into play. Think of it as a visual diary, a timeline that captures your evolution throughout the 28-Day Wall Pilates Program. It's a tangible reflection of your determination, effort, and progress, offering a clear snapshot of your journey.

Crafting Your Personal Progress Chart

Creating your progress chart can be a fun and creative process. It doesn't have to be fancy or elaborate; a simple chart on a piece of paper works just fine. The key is to make it personal and meaningful to you.

Now, think about what you want to track on this chart. It could be the number of reps for specific exercises, the duration of your Wall Plank, the flexibility improvements in your Wall Roll Down, or any other aspect of your Wall Pilates practice. Write these parameters on your chart.

The Power of Visualization in Motivating Progress

Every day after your workout, take a few minutes to update your progress chart. Fill in the number of reps you did, the duration of your plank, or any other measure you're tracking. Use colors, stickers, or symbols to make it visually appealing.

Seeing your progress visualized on the chart can be incredibly motivating. It's a reminder of how far you've come, a celebration of your achievements, and a catalyst for your future progress. On days when you're feeling low or unmotivated, glance at your progress chart. It's a visual pep talk, a statement that says, "Look at what you've achieved. You can do this!"

A Progress Chart: More Than Just Numbers

While your progress chart tracks measurable aspects of your Wall Pilates practice, it also tells a deeper, more personal story. It's not just about the numbers; it's about the effort behind those numbers, the commitment, the sweat, the moments of triumph, and even the moments of struggle.

Your progress chart is a testament to your Wall Pilates journey. It's a reflection of your dedication, resilience, and growth. It's a narrative of transformation, one day, one workout, one rep at a time. So, as you fill in your chart each day, remember to look beyond the numbers. See the journey, see the transformation, see the power and potential within you.

Congratulations on completing your progress chart. This simple tool, filled with numbers and colors, holds a profound message - a message of strength, determination, and progress. It's a symbol of your Wall Pilates journey, a testament to your commitment, and a beacon guiding you towards your goals. And though you've reached the end of this section, remember that this is not an end. It's a milestone on your ongoing journey, a journey of strength, flexibility, and holistic wellness—one that continues to unfold with each Wall Pilates workout, each day, each breath. So keep going, keep growing, and keep charting your progress. Your Wall Pilates adventure is only just getting started.

Celebrating Your Achievements. Recognizing Small Wins

Success isn't always about grand achievements and monumental feats. Sometimes, it's about the small wins, the seemingly insignificant victories that pave the way to your ultimate goals. In the realm of Wall Pilates, these small wins could be anything from holding your Wall Plank a few seconds longer, executing a Wall Push-Up with perfect form, or even simply completing your workout when you didn't really feel like it.

What matters is that you acknowledge these wins. Take a moment after each workout to reflect on what you achieved. Congratulate yourself for pushing through challenges, for showing up, and for moving your body in ways that serve your health and well-being. These small wins are worth celebrating; they are the stepping stones leading you towards your larger goals.

Rewarding Consistency

In Wall Pilates, as in life, consistency is key. It's not about doing a lot in a short time; it's about doing a little, consistently, over a long period. It's about showing up for your workouts, day after day, week after week. It's about making Wall Pilates a part of your lifestyle, a habit that nurtures your body and mind.

Rewarding yourself for this consistency can be a powerful motivator. It could be as simple as treating yourself to a relaxing bubble bath after a week of regular workouts, buying that new workout outfit you've been eyeing after a month of consistency, or even taking a well-deserved rest day. These rewards bring joy and reinforce your commitment to staying consistent with your Wall Pilates practice.

Reflecting on the Journey

As you progress through your Wall Pilates practice, it's essential to pause and reflect on your journey - the progress you've made, the challenges you've overcome, and the changes you've noticed in your body and mind.

This reflection is not just about acknowledging your physical progress; it's also about recognizing your mental and emotional growth. Are you more mindful of your body and its movements? Do you feel more connected to your breath? Has your stress level decreased? Are you more confident and more comfortable in your own skin?

As you reflect, remember to be kind to yourself. Every body is unique, and changes happen at different rates. Celebrate your progress, no matter how small it may seem. Know that with each Wall Roll Down, each Wall Push-Up, and each Wall Squat, you are nurturing your health, strengthening your body, and empowering your spirit.

So here you are, standing tall and strong, not just against your wall but also in your life. You've set your goals, followed the program, tracked your progress, and celebrated your achievements. You've not just worked out; you've worked in, cultivating strength, flexibility, and balance from the inside out. This is the power of Wall Pilates, the power of you. And while your 28-day program may be coming to an end, your Wall Pilates adventure continues. Because Wall Pilates is not just a fitness regimen; it's a lifestyle, a commitment to your health and wellbeing. So, keep going, keep growing, and keep celebrating your achievements. You've got this!

Elevating Your Practice: Basic to Intermediate Wall Pilates

Like a book you can't put down or a song you can't stop humming, Wall Pilates has a way of captivating you. Its unique blend of simplicity, challenge, and effectiveness makes it a practice that you want to delve deeper into. But how do you take your practice to the next level? How do you progress from basic to intermediate Wall Pilates? Let's find out!

Taking Your Practice to the Next Level

Progression from Basic to Intermediate: The Stepping Stones

Picture yourself learning a new language. You start with the basics - the alphabet, some common phrases, basic grammar rules. As you become comfortable with these, you start forming sentences, learning more complex words, and understanding the nuances of the language. The world of Wall Pilates is no different.

You've got the basics down - the Wall Stand, the Wall Roll Down, the Wall Push-Up. Now, it's time to start forming 'sentences', combining these basic 'words' into a flowing, dynamic practice. This involves learning new exercises, understanding their mechanics, and incorporating them into your routine.

So, how do you make this progression? It's all about stepping outside your comfort zone, one step at a time. You could add a new exercise to your routine each week. Or, you could challenge yourself by adding more reps or holding each position for a bit longer. Remember, it's not about making a big leap but taking small, consistent steps towards progression.

Importance of Consistency: The Key to Progression

Imagine planting a seed in your garden. You water it regularly, ensure it gets enough sunlight, and it grows into a beautiful plant over time. Your Wall Pilates practice is like that seed. With consistent practice, it can grow and flourish, significantly improving your strength, flexibility, and overall fitness.

Consistency means showing up for your workouts, even on busy days, even when you don't feel like it. It means sticking to your workout schedule three or more times a week or every day. It means pushing through the challenges, celebrating the wins, and staying committed to your practice, no matter what.

Listening to Your Body: Your Inner Guide

In the hustle and bustle of life, we often forget to listen to our bodies. We push through fatigue, ignore discomfort, and often end up doing more harm than good. In Wall Pilates, listening to your body is crucial, especially as you progress from basic to intermediate.

Your body is your best guide. It tells you when to push harder and when to ease off. It tells you which exercises work best for you and which ones you need to modify. It even tells you when to rest and recover. All you need to do is listen.

So, as you embark on this new phase of your Wall Pilates practice, remember to tune into your body. Pay attention to how it feels during and after each workout. Notice any discomfort, tightness, or fatigue. Use these signals to tailor your practice, ensuring it's not only effective but also safe and enjoyable.

So, there you have it - your roadmap to progressing from basic to intermediate Wall Pilates. Remember, progression is a personal journey. It's not about how quickly you can learn a new exercise or how many reps you can do. It's about improving at your own pace, challenging your limits, and celebrating your progress. So, take it one step at a time, enjoy the journey, and look forward to the exciting challenges and achievements ahead.

Chapter 8: Challenging Moves for Core Strength

Wall Mountain Climbers: Scaling Heights of Core Power

Imagine standing at the foot of a towering mountain, ready to conquer the peak. Now, transpose that image to your Wall Pilates practice. Meet the Wall Mountain Climbers, an exercise that's as challenging as it sounds but also incredibly effective in strengthening your core, improving your cardiovascular fitness, and boosting your overall stamina.

Start by getting into the Wall Plank position, hands on the wall and body forming a straight line. Now, begin your climb. Bend one knee and draw it towards your chest. Return it to the starting position and repeat the movement with the other knee. Keep alternating legs, just like you're climbing a mountain.

As you perform the Wall Mountain Climbers, engage your core and maintain a steady rhythm. Each knee drive is a step higher on your mountain, each breath a gust of fresh, invigorating mountain air.

Wall Plank Knee Tucks: Amplifying Core Engagement

Next up on our list of core-challenging exercises are the Wall Plank Knee Tucks. They are a fantastic way to target your abs, obliques, and lower back, all while improving your balance and coordination.

Begin in your Wall Plank position, body straight and core engaged. Now, add a twist to your climb. Bend one knee and bring it sideways towards your elbow. Return it to the starting position and repeat with the other knee. Keep alternating sides, tucking your knees as close to your elbows as you can.

Remember to keep your movements controlled and your body stable, resisting the urge to sway from side to side. Each knee tuck brings a wave of engagement through your core, a ripple of strength that reaffirms your power.

Wall Plank Jacks: A Full-Body Challenge

Finally, let's take on the Wall Plank Jacks, an advanced exercise that's set to get your heart pumping, your muscles working, and your body radiating with energy.

Kickstart this move from your trusty Wall Plank position. Now, instead of climbing or tucking, you'll be jumping. Like a traditional jumping jack, jump your feet out to the sides and back together. Keep your core tight and maintain the alignment of your body as you perform the jumps.

The Wall Plank Jacks are a core exercise and a full-body challenge. They work your arms, shoulders, chest, abs, obliques, back, glutes, and legs in one dynamic move. Plus, the jumping action gets your heart rate up, making this a fantastic cardio exercise too.

As you explore these challenging moves, remember to be patient with yourself. They might seem difficult at first, but you'll get the hang of it with practice. And remember, each Wall Mountain Climber, each Wall Plank Knee Tuck, and each Wall Plank Jack is a testament to your strength, your resilience, and your progress. So, embrace the challenge, trust your strength, and keep climbing towards your fitness peak.

Enhancing Flexibility and Balance: The Dual Pillars of Wall Pilates

Wall Splits: Stretching Your Limits

Let's initiate this exploration with Wall Splits, a potent move that stretches your hamstrings, opens up your hips, and enhances your lower body flexibility.

To get started, position yourself close to the wall, lying on your back. Extend one leg up the wall while the other stays flat on the floor, forming an "L" shape. Gradually slide the foot on the floor towards the wall, trying to form a split. Keep both legs as straight and relaxed as possible.

As you perform the Wall Splits, pay attention to your breathing. Inhale to prepare, and exhale as you slide into the split, allowing your breath to guide your movement. Remember, the goal isn't to force your legs into a perfect split but rather to gently stretch your muscles and improve flexibility over time.

Wall Scissors: Fine-Tuning Your Flexibility

Next, we have Wall Scissors, an exercise that enhances flexibility, strengthens your core, and improves balance.

Starting in a similar position as the Wall Splits, extend one leg up the wall while the other stays flat on the floor. Now, engage your core and lift the lower leg off the floor, bringing it as close to the other leg as possible. Lower it down and repeat.

As you perform the Wall Scissors, focus on maintaining control and stability. This exercise isn't about speed or how high you can lift your leg; it's about moving with precision and control, challenging your balance, and enhancing your flexibility.

Wall Arabesque: Balancing Grace and Strength

Lastly, let's explore the Wall Arabesque, a beautiful and challenging exercise that tests your balance, strengthens your core, and stretches your body.

Begin by standing a foot away from the wall, facing away. Lean forward and place your hands on the wall, coming into an inclined position. Now, engage your core and lift one leg off the floor, extending it behind you. Keep your body straight and your leg as high as possible.

As you perform the Wall Arabesque, focus on maintaining balance and control. Feel your supporting leg rooting into the ground, your core stabilizing your body, and your extended leg reaching towards the sky. This exercise is a testament to the power of Wall Pilates, combining grace, strength, and balance in one dynamic move.

Flexibility and balance are two key elements of Wall Pilates. They allow you to perform each exercise with ease, control, and precision. Incorporating exercises like Wall Splits, Wall Scissors, and Wall Arabesque into your routine can enhance these vital skills and elevate your Wall Pilates practice.

Remember, Wall Pilates is not a race or a competition. It's a personal journey towards better health and wellbeing. So, take your time with these exercises, listen to your body, and most importantly, enjoy the process. With patience, consistency, and a positive mindset, you'll see improvements in your flexibility and balance and experience the many benefits of Wall Pilates.

So, here's to your Wall Pilates practice - a practice of strength, flexibility, balance, and endless possibilities. A practice that challenges you, empowers you, and helps you become the best version of yourself. Keep going, keep growing, and keep discovering the magic of Wall Pilates. Your adventure is only just getting started.

Maintaining Focus and Control: The Inner Game of Wall Pilates
Breathing Techniques: The Life Force of Your Practice

Let's start by breathing life into our practice. In Wall Pilates, each inhalation and exhalation is not merely a physiological process but an integral part of your movements. Each breath you take fuels your exercises, deepens your stretches, and propels your progress.

To harness the power of your breath, incorporate specific breathing techniques into your practice. Start with lateral breathing, a Pilates-specific technique that involves inhaling deeply into the sides and back of your rib cage. As you inhale, feel your rib cage expand laterally, like an accordion opening up. As you exhale, contract your ribs and engage your core.

Another effective technique is paced breathing. This involves syncing your breath with your movements. For instance, you could inhale as you slide into a Wall Squat and exhale as you rise up. This paced breathing enhances your performance and promotes mindfulness, keeping you present and focused in your practice.

Breathing, as simple as it may seem, is the life force of your Wall Pilates practice. It brings energy, rhythm, and focus to your workouts. So, make every breath count. Fill your lungs with air, your movements with energy, and your practice with life.

Mind-Body Connection: Uniting the Physical and the Mental

Next, let's delve into the realm of the mind-body connection, a fascinating aspect of Wall Pilates that sets it apart from traditional workouts. Wall Pilates is not just about moving your body; it's about syncing your movements with your mind, creating a harmonious symphony of physical action and mental focus.

Cultivating a strong mind-body connection starts with mindfulness - being fully present in each moment, each breath, and each movement. As you perform your Wall Pilates exercises, tune into your body. Feel your muscles contracting and relaxing, your heart beating, your breath flowing. Notice the subtleties of each movement, the nuances of each transition, the rhythm of your routine.

This heightened awareness improves your performance and deepens your Wall Pilates experience. It turns your workout into a moving meditation, a space where you can connect with your body, calm your mind, and recharge your spirit.

Overcoming Plateaus: Embracing Challenges and Celebrating Progress

Lastly, let's talk about plateaus, a common phenomenon in any fitness journey. A plateau is a stage where you stop seeing progress despite consistent efforts. While it can be disheartening, it's important to remember that plateaus are a normal part of the process. They signify that your body has adapted to the current level of challenge and is ready for more.

You should shake things up a bit to overcome plateaus in your Wall Pilates practice. Try new exercises, add more reps or sets, or increase the intensity of your workouts. Challenge yourself, but do so with respect for your body's limits.

And most importantly, celebrate your progress. Every Wall Push-Up, every Wall Plank, and every Wall Squat is a testament to your strength, resilience, and commitment. Every workout brings you one step closer to your fitness goals and one step further on your path to health and well-being.

So, there you have it - the inner game of Wall Pilates. From the life-giving power of your breath to the unity of your mind and body, from the challenges of plateaus to the triumphs of progress, this is what Wall Pilates is all about. It's more than just a workout; it's a practice of self-discovery, self-improvement, and self-celebration. And with each breath, each movement, each moment, you're not just working out; you're working in, cultivating a stronger, healthier, and happier you.

Now, as we wrap up this chapter, know that the journey doesn't end here. Wall Pilates is a lifelong practice, a constant learning and growth journey. So keep breathing, moving, exploring, and most importantly, enjoying your Wall Pilates practice. Your adventure is only just beginning. Let's continue our exploration in the next chapter, where we'll dive into the exciting world of personalized routines and modifications in Wall Pilates. See you there!

Chapter 9: Turning Up the Heat: From Intermediate to Advanced Wall Pilates

Welcome to the exhilarating terrain of advanced Wall Pilates! Think about the thrill of completing a complex puzzle, hitting a high note in your favorite song, or finally perfecting that intricate recipe. That's the same exhilaration you'll experience as you venture into the realm of advanced Wall Pilates.

You've laid a solid foundation with basic and intermediate moves, and now it's time to push your boundaries, test your limits, and unveil the full potential of your strength and flexibility. But don't worry, we're in this together. With a focus on safety and a spirit of exploration, let's dive deeper into the transformative world of Wall Pilates.

Pushing Your Boundaries - Embracing Challenges

Imagine standing on a diving board, looking down at the sparkling water below. It's a bit scary, a bit exciting. You take a deep breath, gather your courage, and jump. The moment you hit the water, you realize it wasn't as scary as you thought. In fact, it was exhilarating.

That's what embracing challenges in Wall Pilates is like. It might seem daunting at first, but once you take the leap, you discover a world of strength and flexibility you never knew existed.

Advanced Wall Pilates moves are challenging, yes, but they are also incredibly rewarding. They push you out of your comfort zone, helping you uncover new layers of strength, flexibility, and resilience.

So, don't shy away the next time you encounter a challenging move. Instead, embrace it. Remember, every challenge is an opportunity to learn, grow, and transform.

Overcoming Fear of Advanced Moves

Fear is a natural reaction when faced with something new or challenging. It's your body's way of saying, "Hey, this is unfamiliar. Be careful." But while it's important to listen to your body, it's equally important not to let fear hold you back.

Think about learning to ride a bike. At first, it was scary. You were afraid of falling, of getting hurt. But with practice, you learned to balance, to pedal, to steer. And before you knew it, you were zooming around with a big grin on your face.

Overcoming fear of advanced Wall Pilates moves is a lot like learning to ride a bike. It starts with understanding the move. Break it down step by step, visualize it, practice it in your mind. Then, try it out slowly, carefully, without rushing. Use modifications if needed, and always prioritize proper form and alignment.

With time, patience, and practice, you'll find that the moves you once feared are now part of your regular routine. And who knows, they might even become your favorites!

Importance of Rest and Recovery

Just as a car needs regular tune-ups to run smoothly, your body needs regular rest and recovery to perform at its best. In the world of advanced Wall Pilates, rest and recovery are not just important - they are essential.

Rest days give your body the time it needs to repair and rebuild muscle tissue, which can lead to increased strength and improved performance. They also give you a much-needed mental break, allowing you to come back to your workouts refreshed and rejuvenated.

On the other hand, recovery is about what you do after your workouts to help your body heal and bounce back. This could include stretching, foam rolling, hydrating, eating nutrient-rich foods, and getting enough sleep.

So, as you push your boundaries in advanced Wall Pilates, remember to balance your efforts with adequate rest and recovery. Because taking care of your body isn't just about working out - it's also about resting, recovering, and respecting your body's needs.

High Intensity, High Reward Moves: Embrace the Challenge

Wall Handstand: Inversion Innovation

Feeling brave? Let's start with the Wall Handstand, an inversion that defies gravity and excitingly challenges your body. This move works your entire body, particularly your shoulders, arms, and core.

To perform a Wall Handstand, face the wall and place your hands on the floor about a foot away from the wall. Kick one leg up towards the wall, followed by the other leg. Aim to get your body in a straight line, with your hands directly under your shoulders. Hold this position for a few breaths, engaging your core and pushing the floor away with your hands.

A word of caution: The Wall Handstand is a challenging move that requires

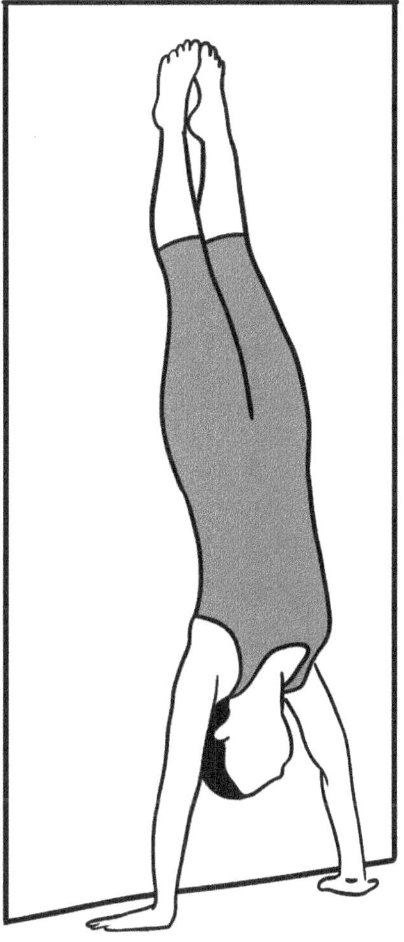

Wall Handstand

strength, balance, and confidence. Don't rush into it. Take your time, practice regularly, and gradually work your way up to the full handstand.

Wall Pike: Core Control at its Peak

Next up is the Wall Pike, a powerful exercise that targets your core and challenges your upper body strength. It's like an elevated plank that takes your Wall Pilates practice to new heights.

Engage your core and slowly start to walk your feet up the wall, keeping your legs straight. At the same time, walk your hands towards the wall, maintaining a strong plank position. Go as high as you feel comfortable, aiming to get your body into an inverted "V" shape.

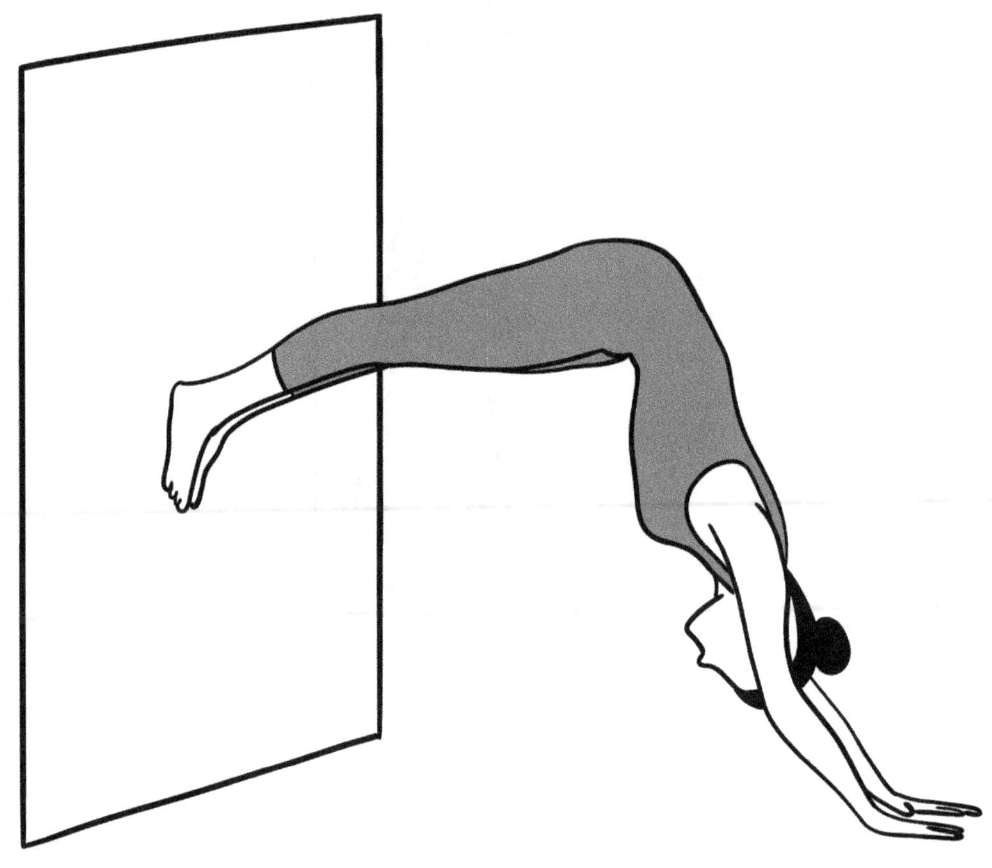

Wall Pike

The Wall Pike is a testament to your power and control. Each step you take up the wall brings a wave of engagement through your core, a ripple of strength that reaffirms your power.Wall Side Plank: A Twist on a Classic

Last but not least is the Wall Side Plank, a twist on the classic plank that targets your obliques and enhances your balance.

To perform a Wall Side Plank, start by standing sideways next to the wall. Lean into the wall with your forearm and step your feet out, one in front of the other. Lift your hips to create a straight line from head to heels, just like in a regular plank. For an extra challenge, raise your top arm towards the ceiling.

The Wall Side Plank might seem simple, but it packs a punch. It requires strength, balance, and precision, making it a worthy addition to your advanced Wall Pilates repertoire.

As you explore these high-intensity moves, remember to celebrate your progress. Every handstand, every pike, every side plank is a victory, a symbol of your strength, resilience, and determination. You're not just working out; you're sculpting your body, honing your skills, and cultivating a fitness practice that's uniquely yours. So, embrace the challenge, trust your strength, and keep pushing your boundaries. Your Wall Pilates adventure continues to unfold.

Advanced Techniques for Strength and Flexibility

Wall Bridge: Crafting Stability and Flexibility

The Wall Bridge, a unique take on the classic bridge pose, is a powerful move that targets your glutes, hamstrings, and lower back. This advanced technique enhances strength and promotes flexibility in your hip flexors and chest.

Position yourself on the floor, back down, with your knees bent and feet flat against the wall. Arms rest by your sides, palms facing down. Ignite your core and press into your heels to lift your hips off the floor, reaching towards the ceiling. Your body should form a straight line from your shoulders to your knees. Hold this position for a few seconds, feeling the engagement in your glutes and hamstrings. Then, slowly lower your hips back down to the floor, engaging your core to control the descent.

As you perform the Wall Bridge, focus on maintaining a smooth, controlled movement. It's not about how high you can lift your hips but rather the quality of the lift and the control on the way down.

Wall Single-Leg Squat: Sculpting Strength and Balance

Next up, we have the Wall Single-Leg Squat, an advanced move that takes the traditional squat and adds a twist. This exercise amplifies your lower body strength and requires balance and stability.

Start by standing a foot away from the wall, facing away. Lean your back against the wall for support. Shift your weight onto one foot and lift the other foot off the ground. Maintain your balance as you bend your standing knee, sliding down the wall into a squat. Ensure your knee stays directly over your ankle. Push through your standing foot to rise back up to the starting position.

The Wall Single-Leg Squat can be challenging, but with consistent practice, you'll notice increased strength in your legs and improved balance.

Wall Single-Leg Stretch: Elevating Flexibility and Control
Last on our list of advanced techniques is the Wall Single-Leg Stretch. This exercise offers a deep stretch for your hamstrings while also engaging your core and improving your balance.

Lie on your back with your feet on the wall, knees bent. Engage your core and lift one foot off the wall, extending it towards the ceiling. Grasp the back of your lifted leg at your calf or thigh and gently pull it towards your chest for a deep hamstring stretch. At the same time, press your other foot into the wall for stability.

The Wall Single-Leg Stretch is about reaching your foot to your chest and maintaining control and alignment throughout the exercise. As you stretch your hamstring, keep your hips square, your core engaged, and your neck and shoulders relaxed.

Incorporating these advanced techniques into your Wall Pilates routine will enhance your strength and flexibility and refine your control and balance. As you progress in your practice, remember to listen to your body, honor your limits, and enjoy the process of growth and improvement. The beauty of Wall Pilates lies in the journey, and every step you take is a testament to your commitment, resilience, and strength. So, keep exploring, keep challenging yourself, and keep enjoying the transformative power of Wall Pilates.

Visualizing Success: Illustrations for Advanced Wall Pilates Positions
The Power of Visualization
Imagine you're trying to build a piece of furniture but only have the list of parts and written instructions. Sounds daunting, right? That's where an instruction

manual with clear diagrams comes in handy. The same applies to Wall Pilates. Visualizations, in the form of illustrations or diagrams, can significantly enhance your understanding and execution of the exercises, especially when you're advancing to more complex moves.

As you progress to advanced Wall Pilates exercises, these illustrations serve as a valuable tool to guide your practice. They offer a visual roadmap to correct alignment, form, and technique, helping you perform each exercise safely and effectively. So, as you explore these advanced moves, let these illustrations light your path, enhancing your understanding, boosting your confidence, and inspiring your success.

Mindfulness in Advanced Practice: The Inner Dance of Wall Pilates Incorporating Meditation: The Calm within the Storm

Advanced Wall Pilates is like a dance, a lively symphony of strength, flexibility, and balance. But what if, amidst this symphony, we could find a quiet corner, a place of calm and tranquillity? That's where meditation enters the scene.

Meditation is like an oasis of calm in the bustling city of your Wall Pilates practice. It's a space where you can rest, refocus, and recharge. It's a tool that helps you tune into your body, quieten your mind, and cultivate a more profound sense of awareness.

You can weave meditation into your Wall Pilates practice in many ways. It could be a few moments of quiet breathing at the start of your session, setting the tone for your workout. It could be a brief pause between exercises, allowing you to regroup and refocus. Or it could be a longer meditation at the end of your workout, helping you cool down and reflect on your practice.

Body Awareness Techniques: Listening to Your Body's Symphony

As you venture into advanced Wall Pilates, your body becomes an orchestra, playing a symphony of strength, flexibility, and balance. Each muscle plays a note, each breath sets the rhythm, each movement adds a melody. And you, the conductor, need to listen to, understand, and guide this symphony. That's where body awareness techniques come into play.

Body awareness is about tuning into your body's signals, understanding its language, and responding accordingly. It's about feeling each muscle as it contracts and relaxes, noticing each breath as it flows in and out, and sensing each movement as it unfolds.

You can enhance your body awareness through various techniques. It could be a body scan at the start of your workout, checking in with each part of your body. It could be mindful movement, performing each exercise with full attention and intention. Or it could be proprioception exercises, like balancing on one leg, to help you understand your body's position in space.

Benefits of Mindful Movement: The Mind-Body Ballet

Imagine a ballet performance. The dancers move with such grace and precision, each movement flowing into the next, each gesture full of meaning. That's what mindful movement in Wall Pilates is like. It's a ballet of the mind and body, a dance that brings together strength, flexibility, balance, and awareness.

Practicing mindful movement in Wall Pilates has numerous benefits. It enhances your performance, ensuring each exercise is done with optimal form and technique. It reduces the risk of injury by helping you listen to your body and respect its limits. It boosts your enjoyment of the workout, turning it into a moving meditation.

Most importantly, mindful movement fosters a deeper connection between your mind and body. It's not just about doing a Wall Handstand or a Wall Pike. It's about feeling your muscles work, sensing your balance, breathing in rhythm with your movements. It's about being present in each moment, each breath, each movement.

So, there you have it - the inner dance of advanced Wall Pilates. It's a dance of strength and flexibility, a dance of balance and control, a dance of the mind and body. But most importantly, it's your dance, unique and personal. So, embrace it, enjoy it, and keep dancing!

As we close the curtains on this chapter, remember that the dance doesn't end here. It continues, evolving and expanding with each Wall Pilates session. So, keep exploring, challenging yourself, and dancing your unique dance. Your Wall Pilates adventure is only just beginning, and the stage is set for even more exciting performances. So, take a bow, listen to the applause, and get ready for the next act. The spotlight is on you, and your Wall Pilates performance is about to get even more spectacular. Curtain up!

Chapter 10: Fueling Your Wall Pilates Practice: Nutrition for Optimal Performance

Imagine you've just bought a shiny, new sports car. It's sleek, powerful, and built for speed. Now, what type of fuel would you put into this high-performance machine? Would you opt for the cheapest, lowest-quality option? Of course not! You'd choose the best quality fuel because you know that what you put into your car directly impacts its performance.

In many ways, our bodies are like that sports car. They are intricate, powerful machines that require the right type of fuel to perform optimally. This is especially true when it comes to Wall Pilates. Your performance, progress, and overall health are influenced mainly by what you eat. That's why understanding the role of nutrition in fitness is crucial.

The Role of Nutrition in Fitness. Importance of Balanced Diet.

Just as your car needs the right balance of oil, water, and fuel, your body needs a balanced diet to function correctly. Think of a balanced diet as your body's maintenance routine. It's what keeps your engine running smoothly, your parts in good condition, and your performance at its peak.

A balanced diet provides all the nutrients your body needs in the proper proportions. This includes macronutrients (proteins, carbohydrates, and fats), micronutrients (vitamins and minerals), and fiber. It's about variety, moderation, and balance.

For instance, having a colorful salad for lunch, packed with leafy greens, bright vegetables, lean protein, and a handful of nuts, offers a range of nutrients that fuel your body for your afternoon Wall Pilates session.

Role of Macronutrients

If we continue with the car analogy, macronutrients are the main fuel types your car needs: petrol, oil, and coolant. Each plays a unique role in keeping your car running smoothly.

- **Proteins** are the building blocks of your body. They're essential for repairing and building tissues, including the muscles you work so hard during your Wall Pilates sessions. Protein sources include lean meats, fish, eggs, dairy products, legumes, and nuts.

- **Carbohydrates** are your body's main source of energy. They're like the petrol that keeps your engine running. During digestion, carbohydrates are broken down into glucose, which is used to fuel your cells. Sources of healthy carbohydrates include whole grains, fruits, vegetables, and legumes.

- **Fats are a concentrated source of energy**. They're like the oil that keeps your engine lubricated. While fats have often been demonized in the world of dieting, your body needs certain fats for energy and to absorb vitamins. Healthy fats can be found in foods like avocados, olives, nuts, seeds, and fatty fish.

Significance of Micronutrients

Finally, micronutrients are like your car's small but essential parts - the spark plugs, the filters, the battery. You might not notice them much, but your car wouldn't run well without them.

Micronutrients, including vitamins and minerals, play a huge role in many bodily functions. They're involved in everything from energy production to bone health to immunity.

For example, calcium, a mineral, is needed for muscle function and bone health - both crucial for your Wall Pilates practice. Vitamin C, on the other hand, is essential for collagen production, which helps with tissue repair and recovery after a tough workout.

Just as you would take your car for regular tune-ups to keep it running smoothly, nourishing your body with a balanced diet is crucial for optimizing your Wall Pilates practice and overall health. By understanding the role of nutrition in fitness, you can make informed choices that fuel your body for success. After all, a well-fueled body is a well-functioning body, ready to take on the challenge of Wall Pilates and enjoy the journey of health and well-being. So, fill up your tank with nutritional goodness and get ready to power through your Wall Pilates sessions!

Foods to Fuel Your Pilates Practice

Protein-Rich Foods: Building Blocks of Strength

So, let's start with protein, the star player in muscle repair and growth. When you engage in Wall Pilates, your muscles go through a process of breakdown and repair. This cycle is completely normal and is actually how muscles get stronger. Protein is a key component of this process.

Imagine a construction site. Protein is like the bricks that builders use to construct a building. In the same way, your body uses protein to repair damaged muscle fibers and build new ones. This process of muscle protein synthesis is what leads to muscle growth and strength gains.

Moreover, protein can help curb hunger by keeping you fuller for longer. This can be especially useful if you're trying to maintain or lose weight.

So, where can you get your protein? Good sources include lean meats like chicken and turkey, fish like salmon and tuna, and plant-based sources like lentils, chickpeas, and tofu. Eggs and dairy products like Greek yogurt and cottage cheese are also excellent choices.

Complex Carbohydrates: Your Body's Fuel

Next on the list are carbohydrates, the primary source of energy for your body. When you eat carbs, your body breaks them down into glucose, feeling your cells and keeping you going.

Picture a coal-powered train. The coal is burned to produce energy, which powers the train and keeps it moving. Carbohydrates are like the coal for your body—they're burned to produce energy, powering your Wall Pilates workouts and keeping you moving.

However, not all carbohydrates are created equal. While simple carbs like sugar and white bread can provide quick energy, they can also lead to a crash later. On the other hand, complex carbohydrates are digested more slowly, providing a steady, sustained release of energy.

Good sources of complex carbs include whole grains like brown rice, quinoa, and whole-grain bread. Fruits and vegetables are also excellent sources, packed with added bonuses like fiber, vitamins, and minerals.

Healthy Fats: The Unsung Heroes

Lastly, we have fats, the unsung heroes of a balanced diet. Despite what you might've heard, fats are not the enemy. In fact, certain types of fat are essential for your health and can actually support your Wall Pilates practice.

Think of fats as the oil in a car. They keep things running smoothly. Dietary fats support numerous functions in the body, from absorbing vitamins to providing long-lasting energy.

The key is to focus on healthy fats, mainly unsaturated fats. These fats, which are liquid at room temperature, are beneficial for heart health and inflammation. Sources include avocados, nuts and seeds, oily fish like salmon and mackerel, and oils like olive oil and canola oil.

Incorporating these nutrient-dense foods into your diet can fuel your Wall Pilates practice and support your overall health. So, next time you're planning your meals, remember the importance of protein, carbs, and healthy fats. Your body—and your Wall Pilates practice—will thank you.

Meal Planning for Success. Sample Meal Plans.

Imagine you're an artist with a blank canvas in front of you. The canvas is your day, and the meals and snacks you choose are the colors you'll use to create your masterpiece. Each meal is an opportunity to nourish your body, fuel your Wall Pilates practice, and create a colorful, balanced picture of health.

To kick-start your day, how about a protein-packed breakfast? Think Greek yoghurt topped with berries and a sprinkle of chia seeds or scrambled eggs with spinach and whole grain toast. This meal sets the tone for the day, providing you with the energy to dive into your Wall Pilates routine.

For lunch, consider a vibrant salad with lean protein like grilled chicken or chickpeas, a rainbow of vegetables, and healthy fat like avocado or olive oil. This nutrient-dense meal will keep you fueled throughout the afternoon.

When it's time for dinner, fill half your plate with colorful vegetables, a quarter with lean protein like fish or tofu, and a quarter with complex carbohydrates like quinoa or sweet potato. This visually balanced plate ensures you're getting a good mix of nutrients to support your recovery and prepare you for the next day's Wall Pilates session.

And don't forget about snacks! A handful of nuts, a piece of fruit, or some carrot sticks with hummus can keep your energy levels steady between meals.

Remember, these meal plans are just a guide. Feel free to mix, match, swap ingredients, and adjust portions to suit your unique needs and preferences. The goal is to create a meal plan that you enjoy that fuels your body and supports your Wall Pilates practice.

Importance of Meal Timing

Just as timing is crucial in a Wall Pilates workout, it's also key when it comes to nutrition. When you eat can be just as important as what you eat.

Eating breakfast can kick-start your metabolism and give you the energy for your morning Wall Pilates session. Try not to skip this meal, even if you're not a big breakfast eater. Even a small, nutrient-dense meal can make a difference.

Lunch and dinner should ideally be spaced about four to five hours apart, with a small snack in between if needed. This timing helps keep your energy levels stable and prevents overeating at meal times.

As for pre- and post-workout meals, aim to eat a balanced meal or snack one to two hours before your Wall Pilates session. This gives your body enough time to digest and use the nutrients for energy. After your workout, try to eat within an hour to replenish your energy stores and aid in muscle recovery.

Everyone's body is different, so what works for one person may not work for another. Listen to your body's hunger and fullness cues, and adjust your meal timing accordingly.

Tips for Healthy Snacking

When it comes to snacking, it's easy to reach for the nearest bag of chips or a chocolate bar. But with a bit of planning, you can turn snack time into another opportunity to nourish your body.

First, think of snacks as mini-meals. They should contain a balance of macronutrients - protein, carbohydrates, and fats - just like your main meals. This could be as simple as an apple with a handful of nuts or some whole-grain crackers with cheese.

Second, aim for whole, unprocessed foods whenever possible. These foods are closer to their natural state, which means they're typically higher in nutrients and lower in added sugars and unhealthy fats.

Finally, remember that snacks are meant to tide you over until your next meal, not replace it. Keep your portions small and listen to your hunger cues. If you're not really hungry, you might not need a snack, even if it's 'snack time'.

By incorporating these tips into your routine, you can ensure your snacks are working for you, not against you. They'll provide you with the energy boost you need, without derailing your health and fitness goals. So, next time you feel peckish between meals, reach for a healthy snack and reap the benefits of your Wall Pilates practice.

In conclusion, nutrition plays a vital role in your Wall Pilates journey. By fueling your body with balanced meals, timing your meals to support your energy levels, and choosing healthy snacks, you can enhance your performance, boost your recovery, and feel your best both during and after your workouts. So, raise a glass (of water!) to good nutrition and its incredible power to nourish, fuel, and transform your body, one Wall Pilates workout at a time.

Hydration and Recovery: Quenching the Thirst of Your Body

Importance of Water Intake

Imagine a river flowing freely, its waters clear and sparkling. Now, imagine the same river with its waters depleted. The riverbed is exposed, and the flow is sluggish. Our bodies are much like that river. Water is the lifeline that keeps our systems running smoothly, and when it's in short supply, our performance can suffer.

Water is involved in almost every bodily function. It helps regulate body temperature, lubricates joints, delivers nutrients to cells, and even aids digestion. In your Wall Pilates practice, staying well-hydrated means you can perform at your best, pushing through those challenging exercises and maintaining your stamina throughout your session.

So, how much water should you drink? A good rule of thumb is to drink at least eight glasses (64 ounces) of water a day. However, you might need more if you're sweating heavily during your Wall Pilates workouts. A good indicator of hydration is the color of your urine. If it's light yellow, you're probably well-hydrated. If it's darker, it's time to drink up!

Role of Electrolytes

While water forms the base of your hydration strategy, electrolytes are another key player in the game. These are minerals that carry an electric charge, and they play a crucial role in maintaining fluid balance, nerve function, and muscle contractions.

When you sweat during your Wall Pilates workouts, you lose water and electrolytes, particularly sodium and potassium. Replacing these lost electrolytes is just as important as replacing lost water.

You can replenish electrolytes through your diet. Sodium is found in table salt and many processed foods, while potassium is abundant in fruits and vegetables, especially bananas and oranges. Consider an electrolyte drink for intense workouts or hot weather. Just watch out for high sugar content!

Recovery Foods

After pushing your boundaries in a Wall Pilates session, it's time to refuel your body with recovery foods. These are foods that help replenish your energy stores, repair muscle tissue, and reduce inflammation.

First on the list are proteins, the building blocks of muscle. Consuming protein after your workout can help repair and grow your muscles. Think Greek yogurt, a protein shake, or a chicken breast.

Next up are carbohydrates. Your body uses carbs for energy, and your carb stores are depleted after a workout. Replenishing these stores can speed up recovery and prepare you for your next workout. Opt for complex carbs like whole grains, fruits, and vegetables.

Lastly, don't forget about antioxidants. These compounds help reduce inflammation and speed up recovery. Berries, cherries, and leafy green vegetables are all rich in antioxidants.

So, there you have it. Hydration and recovery are key components of your Wall Pilates practice. By drinking enough water, replenishing electrolytes, and nourishing your body with recovery foods, you're setting the stage for optimal performance and progress. It's another step towards turning your Wall Pilates sessions into a well-oiled, high-performing routine. And with that, you're ready to move on to the next phase of your Wall Pilates adventure! So, grab your water bottle, have a bite of that protein bar, and let's continue to explore the transformative power of Wall Pilates.

Chapter 11: Adapting Wall Pilates for Every Stage of Life

Picture this: the sun is setting, casting a beautiful, golden glow on a lively park scene. There's a group of elderly folks laughing and chatting as they gracefully move their bodies in unison against a park wall. A little further off, you see a group of children mimicking the adults, their faces filled with joy and curiosity. On the other hand, a group of teenagers are engrossed in their own wall Pilates session, their faces reflecting focus and determination. This beauty of Wall Pilates transcends age, embracing everyone from children to seniors, creating a community bound by the shared love for this holistic practice.

In this chapter, we will explore how Wall Pilates can be adapted to different stages of life, starting with the golden years. Wall Pilates offers a wealth of benefits for seniors, from enhancing bone health to improving balance and flexibility. Its gentle yet effective exercises provide a safe and enjoyable way for seniors to stay active and maintain their health and well-being.

Wall Pilates for Senior - Benefits for Bone Health

As we age, our bone health naturally decreases, increasing the risk of conditions such as osteoporosis. With its weight-bearing exercises, Wall Pilates offers an effective strategy to combat this issue. Engaging in weight-bearing exercises like the Wall Squat or Wall Push-Up encourages our body to produce more bone cells, leading to stronger and denser bones.

Enhancing Flexibility

Flexibility can also decline with age, leading to stiffness and reduced range of motion. This is where Wall Pilates shines. With exercises like the Wall Roll Down and Wall Leg Slides, seniors can gently stretch their muscles and increase their flexibility. This improves their mobility and enhances their quality of life, making daily activities easier and more enjoyable.

Improving Balance and Stability

One of the most significant benefits of Wall Pilates for seniors is its ability to improve balance and stability. Falling is a common concern among seniors, and improving balance is a key preventive measure. For instance, the Wall Plank and Wall Mountain Climbers require the engagement of the core muscles, the powerhouse of our body, which plays a critical role in maintaining balance and stability.

Incorporating these exercises into a regular routine can help seniors enhance their balance, strengthen their core, and ultimately increase their confidence and independence.

For seniors to engage in Wall Pilates safely and effectively, it's crucial to keep the following tips in mind:

Tips for Seniors

- Start Slow and Steady: Seniors new to Wall Pilates should start with basic exercises and gradually progress to more challenging ones as their strength and flexibility improve.

- Listen to Your Body: It's essential to pay attention to how your body feels during the exercises. If an exercise causes discomfort or pain, stop and rest.

- Stay Hydrated: Drinking plenty of water during the workouts is crucial to prevent dehydration.

- Use a Mat: Use a mat or a soft rug to provide cushioning and prevent slips during the exercises.

- **Consult a Physician: Always consult with a healthcare provider before starting any new exercise program.**

Implementing these guidelines can help seniors enjoy the benefits of Wall Pilates safely and effectively, improving their overall health, well-being, and quality of life. So, to all the seniors out there, it's never too late to start your Wall Pilates journey. Get ready to embrace a healthier, happier, and more active lifestyle with Wall Pilates!

Introducing Children to Wall Pilates - Making Workouts Fun

Imagine a playground. Children are swinging, sliding, climbing, and laughing. They're having fun. Yes, but they're also building strength, coordination, and balance. This is the essence of Wall Pilates for children. It's about introducing physical activity in a playful and enjoyable way.

Think of the Wall Stand as an invisible chair game or the Wall Squat as a mimic of a frog's leap. By turning exercises into games, we can engage children in Wall Pilates and make their workouts enjoyable.

Remember, fun is a powerful motivator, especially for kids. When they associate Wall Pilates with fun, they're more likely to stick with it and look forward to their workouts.

Encouraging Regular Physical Activity

In a world dominated by screens, getting children to engage in regular physical activity can be a challenge. With its unique and exciting exercises, Wall Pilates provides a wonderful solution.

The beauty of Wall Pilates is that it doesn't require any special equipment or a large space. Kids can practice Wall Push-Ups or Wall Planks in their bedrooms, living rooms, or even outdoors against a safe wall. This accessibility makes it easier for kids to incorporate Wall Pilates into their daily routines.

By encouraging regular physical activity from an early age, we set children on a path to a healthier lifestyle. Wall Pilates becomes a stepping stone, instilling the habit of movement and the love for fitness.

Building Strength and Coordination

As children grow, their bodies are constantly changing and developing. Wall Pilates can play a pivotal role in this developmental stage by building strength and enhancing coordination.

Exercises like the Wall Plank or Wall Mountain Climbers are excellent for developing core strength. A strong core forms the foundation for overall body strength and is crucial for posture, balance, and athletic performance.

Coordination, on the other hand, is the ability to use different parts of the body smoothly and efficiently. Wall Pilates, with its variety of exercises, helps children improve their body awareness and coordination.

For instance, in the Wall Angel exercise, kids need to move their arms up and down while keeping their back and arms in contact with the wall. This strengthens their upper body and improves their body awareness and coordination.

In a nutshell, introducing Wall Pilates to children presents a unique opportunity. It's about making workouts fun, encouraging regular physical activity, and building strength and coordination. It's about giving children a tool to foster their physical development and instill a lifelong love for fitness.

Wall Pilates for Teens: A Focus on Mind-Body Balance

As a teenager navigating the tumultuous tide of adolescence, Wall Pilates presents an oasis of calm, control, and confidence. The changes both within and around can sometimes seem overwhelming - academic pressures, social dynamics, physical transformations, and budding independence. Amidst all this, establishing a mind-body balance becomes not just beneficial but pivotal.

Stress Management

Picture yourself standing in the eye of a storm, the world whirling in chaos around you. Yet, you remain calm, grounded, and focused. This is the power of stress management - the ability to stay composed in the face of challenges. And Wall Pilates, believe it or not, can be a valuable tool in your stress management kit.

When you're engrossed in a Wall Pilates session, focusing on your breathing and the precision of your movements, the world around you fades away. It's just you and the wall, moving in harmony, existing in the moment. This mindful movement can provide a much-needed break from the daily hustle and bustle, helping you clear your mind and release tension.

Moreover, Wall Pilates is a form of physical activity, and like all physical activities, it triggers the release of endorphins, your body's natural mood boosters. These 'feel-good' hormones can help alleviate stress, promote relaxation, and boost your mood. So, the next time you find stress knocking on your door, turn to your wall and let Wall Pilates wash the worries away.

Building Self-Esteem

Now, let's turn the spotlight on self-esteem, an essential facet of your mental and emotional well-being. Self-esteem is about respecting yourself, acknowledging your worth, and embracing your strengths. And Wall Pilates provides a platform to build and bolster your self-esteem.

Every time you successfully execute a Wall Plank or a Wall Squat, you prove to yourself that you're capable, resilient, and strong. No matter how small, every progression boosts your confidence and reinforces your belief in your abilities. You begin to view yourself not as a teenager grappling with change but as a Wall Pilates practitioner mastering the art of strength, flexibility, and balance.

Moreover, Wall Pilates encourages you to focus on what your body can do rather than how it looks. It shifts the narrative from aesthetic appeal to functional fitness, fostering a positive body image. So, stand tall, stand proud, and let Wall Pilates guide you towards improved self-esteem.

Promoting Healthy Growth

Finally, let's delve into how Wall Pilates can contribute to healthy growth during the teenage years. As your body grows and changes, supporting it with activities that promote strength, flexibility, and overall fitness is crucial. And Wall Pilates fits the bill perfectly.

Wall Pilates targets various muscle groups, promoting balanced muscle development. It encourages flexibility, which is particularly beneficial during growth spurts. It also helps improve posture, an important aspect considering many teenagers' long hours sitting at desks.

Moreover, Wall Pilates is a low-impact activity, which makes it a safe option for teenagers. It's easy on the joints, reducing the risk of injuries.

So, there you have it - Wall Pilates, a practice that transcends the boundaries of age and embraces everyone, from children to seniors. Whether it's enhancing bone health for seniors, making workouts fun for children, or promoting mind-body balance for teens, Wall Pilates offers a multitude of benefits for all ages.

And the beauty of Wall Pilates is that it can be adapted to suit different ages and abilities. With appropriate modifications and safety measures, Wall Pilates can be a safe, effective, and enjoyable activity for everyone. So, no matter your age or fitness level, step up to the wall and experience the transformative power of Wall Pilates for yourself.

Adapting Wall Pilates to Suit You: The Art of Personalization

Modifying Exercises: Tailoring to Your Needs

Imagine you're at a clothing store, trying on a shirt. You love the design, but the fit needs to be corrected. It's too long, too loose. Would you walk away, or would you consider getting it altered? Wall Pilates is similar. Sometimes, an exercise might not be the perfect fit for you. Does that mean you should skip it? Absolutely not! Just like the shirt, exercises can be modified to suit your fit - your body, your comfort, your ability.

Let's take the Wall Plank, for example. Holding a full Wall Plank can be challenging for someone new to Wall Pilates or with wrist discomfort. But it becomes more manageable with a simple modification - doing the plank on the forearms instead of the hands. Similarly, a Wall Squat can be modified by reducing the depth of the squat or using a support for balance.

Modifications aren't a compromise. They're a way to make Wall Pilates work for you. They ensure that every exercise is accessible, doable, and beneficial, irrespective of your age, fitness level, or physical condition.

Ensuring Safety: Your Top Priority

Now, let's talk about safety, a key aspect that must always be at the forefront of your Wall Pilates practice. Think of safety as the seatbelt in your car. It's a non-negotiable, a must-have, a protector.

To ensure safety in Wall Pilates, there are several guidelines to keep in mind. First and foremost, always warm up before starting your workout and cool down afterwards. This helps prepare your body for the workout and gradually brings it back to its normal state afterwards, reducing the risk of injury.

Secondly, maintain proper form and alignment during all exercises. This is not just about effectiveness but also about safety. Incorrect form can lead to strain or injury.

Finally, listen to your body. If an exercise causes pain or discomfort, stop and assess. You may need to adjust your form, modify the exercise, or skip it altogether. Remember, Wall Pilates is about wellness, not pain or harm.

Encouraging Consistency: The Secret Sauce

Let's end this chapter with one last piece of advice: Be consistent. Imagine watering a plant. If you water it regularly, it grows and thrives. But if you water it one day and then forget about it for a week, it struggles to survive. Your Wall Pilates practice is like that plant. It needs regular watering - regular practice - to grow and thrive.

Consistency is the secret sauce to success in Wall Pilates. It's not about doing a two-hour workout one day and then doing nothing for the rest of the week. It's about doing a little bit every day, making Wall Pilates a part of your daily routine.

So, whether it's 10 minutes a day or an hour, morning or evening, at home or in the park, find a routine that works for you and stick to it. And remember, every bit counts. Every Wall Stand, every Wall Push-Up, every Wall Plank brings you one step closer to your fitness goals, one step further on your path to health and well-being.

So, go ahead. Modify your exercises, prioritize your safety, and be consistent. Tailor your Wall Pilates practice to suit your unique needs and abilities. After all, Wall Pilates is not a one-size-fits-all affair. It's a personal journey, a custom-fit practice, a celebration of your individuality. So, embrace it, enjoy it, and make it your own. And remember, the wall is always there, ready to support, challenge, and help you grow. So, step up, take a deep breath, and let's keep exploring the wonderful world of Wall Pilates.

Chapter 12: Embracing the Challenges: Turning Hurdles into Stepping Stones

Imagine you're on a scenic hike. As you navigate the trail, you encounter a series of obstacles - a sudden steep slope, a tricky rock formation, or perhaps a slippery patch of gravel. What do you do? Do you turn back or find a way to overcome these challenges and continue your hike? Like this hike, your Wall Pilates journey may present a few obstacles. But with the right approach, you can transform these challenges into growth, learning, and self-discovery opportunities.

In this chapter, we'll look at some common challenges you might encounter in your Wall Pilates practice and provide practical solutions to help you navigate them. From dealing with time constraints to overcoming plateaus and managing expectations, we'll arm you with the strategies you need to turn these hurdles into stepping stones on your path to health and well-being.

Overcoming Common Challenges - Dealing with Time Constraints

One of the most common challenges in any fitness journey, including Wall Pilates, is finding time for workouts amidst our busy schedules. Finding a spare moment for a workout can often feel like finding a needle in a haystack between work, family commitments, social obligations, and personal chores.

But here's the good news: Wall Pilates is incredibly adaptable and can easily fit into your daily routine. You don't need to dedicate an hour each day; even a few minutes can make a difference. Here are a few practical tips:

- **Early Bird or Night Owl?** Identify your most productive time of the day. Consider a quick Wall Pilates session to kickstart your day if you're a morning person. If you're more energetic in the evenings, unwind with a relaxing workout before bed.

- **Seize the Breaks:** Do you have a few spare minutes during your lunch break or while waiting for dinner to cook? That's a perfect time to squeeze in a quick set of Wall Push-Ups or Wall Planks.

- **TV Time:** Watching your favorite show? Use the ad breaks for a mini Wall Pilates session. Before you know it, you'll have completed a full workout by the end of the episode!

Overcoming Plateaus

Hitting a plateau can be disheartening. This is when you seem to stop making progress despite consistent workouts. But don't be discouraged; plateaus are a normal part of any fitness journey. They're your body's way of saying, "Hey, I need something new!" Here's how to tackle them:

- **Mix It Up:** If you've been doing the same Wall Pilates routine for weeks, it's time to mix things up. Try new exercises, alter the sequence, or adjust the number of sets or reps. Variety will challenge your body in new ways and reignite your progress.

- **Intensity Matters:** Consider increasing the intensity of your workouts. This could mean holding the poses for a few more seconds, adding more repetitions, or incorporating props such as resistance bands for added challenges.

Managing Expectations

It's natural to want quick results in our fast-paced world. But when it comes to Wall Pilates, patience is key. Transforming your body takes time, consistency, and dedication. Here's how to manage your expectations:

- **Realistic Goals:** Set achievable goals for your Wall Pilates practice. Instead of aiming to master a challenging pose in a week, aim to practice it regularly and see how far you get. Remember, it's about progress, not perfection.

- **Celebrate Small Wins:** Did you hold the Wall Plank for a few seconds longer? Did you feel more flexible in the Wall Roll Down? Every improvement, no matter how small, is a victory worth celebrating.

- **Trust the Process:** Wall Pilates is more than just a workout; it's a journey of self-discovery, strength, and wellness. Trust the process, enjoy the trip, and the results will follow.

In the end, remember that each challenge you encounter in your Wall Pilates journey is an opportunity to learn, grow, and become stronger. So, embrace these challenges, harness your inner strength, and keep moving forward. Your

Wall Pilates journey is a testament to your resilience, determination, and the incredible power within you. So, stand tall, breathe deep, and let's continue to conquer these challenges together, one Wall Pilates move at a time.

Building a Regular Pilates Routine - Setting a Schedule

Imagine you're planning a road trip. You map out your route, mark your stops, and schedule your days. It gives you a sense of direction and helps you make the most of your trip. Now, think about your Wall Pilates practice as that road trip. Setting a schedule for your workouts is like mapping out your route. It gives direction to your practice, ensuring you make the most out of your fitness adventure.

Start by looking at your weekly calendar. Identify blocks of free time where you can slot in your Wall Pilates sessions. It could be in the morning before heading to work or in the evenings after you finish your day. The idea is to pick a time when you're most likely to stick to the schedule.

Keep in mind that consistency is critical. Try to slot in your workouts on the same days and times each week. This helps in building a routine and makes it easier to stick to your schedule. Remember, Wall Pilates is your appointment with yourself - make it a priority!

Creating a Dedicated Space

Now, just like you would pack your bags for the road trip, consider creating a dedicated space for your Wall Pilates workouts. Setting aside a specific place for your sessions not only organizes your practice but also enhances your focus and commitment.

Look for a space in your home where you can comfortably perform your Wall Pilates exercises. It could be a corner of your living room, bedroom, or backyard. The key is to find a spot that is quiet, clutter-free and has a sturdy wall.

Once you've identified the space, personalize it. Lay down a comfortable mat, set up a small table or shelf for your water bottle, and add a few motivational quotes or pictures on the wall. The aim is to create a space that inspires you to show up for your practice.

Incorporating Variety

Finally, let's talk about variety. Imagine going on your road trip and seeing the same scenery over and over again. It would get boring, wouldn't it? Just like you would want to explore different routes and stops on your road trip, it's important to incorporate variety in your Wall Pilates routine. Doing so keeps your workouts exciting and challenging.

Experiment with different exercises each week. If you've been doing the Wall Plank regularly, try the Wall Pike. If you've mastered the Wall Squat, challenge yourself with the Wall Mountain Climbers.

You can also play around with your workouts' intensity, duration, and sequence. One day, you go for a high-intensity, short-duration workout, and another day, you opt for a low-intensity, long-duration session. The idea is to keep your body guessing and your mind engaged.

So, there you have it. By setting a schedule, creating a dedicated space, and incorporating variety, you can set yourself up for a successful and enjoyable Wall Pilates routine. It may take planning and organizing, but the rewards are well worth the effort. After all, Wall Pilates isn't just a workout - it's a lifestyle. And these steps can help you make it an integral part of your life. So, plan your schedule, set up your space, and add a dash of variety to your workouts. Your Wall Pilates road trip awaits.

Staying Motivated: Tips from the Pros - Setting Realistic Goals

Imagine you're planning a trip. You wouldn't expect to reach your destination in one giant leap. You plan your route, break down the journey into manageable distances, and take regular pit stops. The same logic applies to your Wall Pilates routine. Setting realistic goals is like plotting your route on the map. It gives you a clear direction and makes your journey manageable and enjoyable.

So, how do you set realistic goals? The key is to keep them specific, measurable, and achievable. For instance, instead of setting a vague goal like "I want to get stronger," try something more specific and measurable, like "I want to hold the Wall Plank for 30 seconds without a break." This gives you a clear target to aim for and makes it easier to track your progress.

Remember, your goals should also be achievable. It's great to aim high, but setting goals that are too ambitious can be demotivating. Start with small, achievable goals, and as you reach them, gradually raise the bar. This way, you're setting yourself up for success and boosting your motivation.

Conclusion - The Takeaways: What We've Learned

Well, my friend, we've come quite a way together on this Wall Pilates journey, haven't we? Let's take a moment to reflect on the valuable lessons we've uncovered.

We've explored the key principles of Wall Pilates, learning how this innovative practice leverages the humble wall to help us build strength, flexibility, and balance. We've discovered how this unique approach to fitness can transform our bodies and minds, bringing us not just physical benefits but mental and emotional ones, too.

Our Wall Pilates practice taught us the importance of consistency and patience. It's not about overnight results or extreme transformations. It's about showing up for ourselves, day after day, and trusting the process.

Equally important, we've delved into the role of nutrition and hydration, understanding how the right fuel can enhance our performance, recovery, and overall well-being. After all, what we put into our bodies is just as important as what we ask our bodies to do.

Your Continued Journey with Wall Pilates

Now, while we're nearing the end of this book, your Wall Pilates journey is far from over. In fact, it's just beginning.

There are numerous advanced techniques for you to explore, each one a new challenge to conquer and a new skill to master. There's always something more to learn, someone new to be inspired by, some new goal to reach for.

Remember, you're not alone in this journey. A vibrant Wall Pilates community is full of fellow enthusiasts who share your passion. So, reach out, connect, and keep the conversation going. We're all here, cheering each other on, learning from one another, and growing together.

A Final Word of Encouragement

As we wrap up, I want to leave you with a few words of encouragement. Embrace the journey, my friend. Celebrate every step forward, every small victory, every bit of progress you make. Remember, it's not about being perfect but being better than you were yesterday.

And most importantly, stay committed to your health and wellbeing. You're worth the effort. You deserve the benefits that Wall Pilates can bring into your life. So, keep showing up for yourself, pushing your limits, and taking care of your body and mind.

Your Next Steps: From Here to Health and Happiness

So, where to from here? Well, that's up to you. You could incorporate Wall Pilates into your daily routine, making it a non-negotiable part of your day. You can share the benefits of Wall Pilates with others, spreading the word and inspiring more people to join the Wall Pilates family. Or you could continue growing and learning, becoming a Wall Pilates instructor yourself.

Whatever path you choose, remember this: Wall Pilates is more than just a workout. It's a lifestyle. It's a commitment to health and happiness. It's a journey of self-discovery, self-improvement, and self-love. So, go forth and conquer, my friend. With Wall Pilates by your side, the world is your oyster. Here's to your health, your happiness, and your continued journey with Wall Pilates!

Make a Difference with Your Review

Review Request:" Wall Pilates for Women: 28-Day Challenge from Beginner to Advanced

How to Share Your Thoughts:
- Visit the Book's Page: Go to the book's page on your preferred platform (Amazon, Goodreads, etc.).
- Compose Your Review: Share what you loved about the book covered.
- Rate the Book: Give it a star rating that reflects your overall impression.

Bonus: The Power of Generosity
As a token of our appreciation, we invite you to consider the power of generosity. Your review helps fellow readers and supports an author who has poured time and expertise into creating this book. Thank you for considering our request. Your generosity in sharing your thoughts can make a world of difference.

With thanks,

Grace Hartley

Skilset Publishing

References

- Wall Pilates Workouts: Effective Techniques For A Stronger Core https://awellnessbody.com/fitness/wall-pilates-workouts-effective-techniques-for-a-stronger-core/

- Physical and psychological benefits of once-a-week Pilates ... https://www.sciencedirect.com/science/article/pii/S0031938416302591

- The Remarkable Health Benefits of Wall Pilates Exercise https://medium.com/@wallpilates/the-remarkable-health-benefits-of-wall-pilates-exercise-ef1eec8901bf

- Real Life Transformations and Success Stories https://wantpilates.com/pilates-before-and-after-real-life-transformations-and-success-stories

- Joseph Pilates https://en.wikipedia.org/wiki/Joseph_Pilates

- The History and Evolution of Classical Pilates: An Overview https://www.sunsetbeachpilates.com/the-history-and-evolution-of-classical-pilates-an-overview-3

- Wall pilates — what to know about 2024's hottest, easiest ... https://nypost.com/2024/01/02/lifestyle/wall-pilates-everything-you-need-to-know-about-the-fitness-trend/

- Fit For The Future: 10 Trends That Will Transform ... https://www.forbes.com/sites/bernardmarr/2023/04/05/fit-for-the-future-10-trends-that-will-transform-the-fitness-industry/

- The Importance of Breathing in Pilates https://www.studiopilates.com/the-importance-of-breathing-in-pilates/

- Pilates Powerhouse – What Does it Mean? https://loveforpilates.com/pilates-powerhouse-mean/

- Doing Pilates The Right Way: Learn The 6 Principles https://pilatesreformersplus.com/blogs/news/doing-pilates-the-right-way-learn-the-6-principles

- How the Pilates Mind-Body Connection Works for You https://www.framefitness.com/blog/news/how-the-pilates-mind-body-connection-works-for-you

- 8 Common Pilates Myths - Busted https://www.thealignmentstudio.com.au/8-common-pilates-myths-busted/

- Why Pilates works in injury rehab and prevention https://us.humankinetics.com/blogs/excerpt/why-pilates-works-in-injury-rehab-and-prevention

- 19 Pilates Benefits Backed By Science https://www.healthline.com/nutrition/pilates-benefits

- Pilates for Overweight or Obesity: A Meta-Analysis - PMC https://www.ncbi.nlm.nih.gov/pmc/articles/PMC7992419/

- Wall Pilates Equipment: Everything You Need To ... https://betterme.world/articles/wall-pilates-equipment/

- How to Create the Best Workout Environment at Home https://www.blog.jetsweatfitness.com/blog-2-1/2021/6/11/how-to-create-the-best-workout-environment-at-home

- 13 Tips for Practicing Pilates Safely at Home https://www.pilateswithamandab.com/post/13-tips-for-practicing-safely-at-home

- How Lighting Changes the Group Fitness Environment https://www.athleticbusiness.com/facilities/fitness/article/15146592/how-lighting-changes-the-group-fitness-environment

- 19 Pilates Benefits Backed By Science https://www.healthline.com/nutrition/pilates-benefits

- Wall Pilates: Effective Exercises That Use Just a Wall https://www.wellandgood.com/wall-pilates/

- The Importance of Good Posture in Pilates https://www.pilatesplatinum.com/importance-good-posture-pilates/

- 10 Essential Pilates Exercises for Core Strength and ... https://www.shantisom.com/en/blog/10-essential-pilates-exercises-for-core-strength-and-flexibility/

- Why 28 Days? The Science Behind Short-Term Fitness ... https://helixsp.com/why-28-days-the-science-behind-short-term-fitness-challenges/

- What Are SMART Fitness Goals? How to Set Them and More https://www.healthline.com/health/fitness/smart-fitness-goals

- How to track your Pilates progress - Pilates Moves You https://pilatesmovesyou.com/how-to-track-your-pilates-progress/

- Celebrating Your Fitness Success https://www.heart.org/en/healthy-living/fitness/staying-motivated/celebrating-your-fitness-success

- Intermediate Wall Pilates Workout 30 min - YouTube https://www.youtube.com/watch?v=yywNPwneVMc

- Pilates Progression: A Whole Person Approach – Part 1 https://thecore.balancedbody.com/pilates-progression-a-whole-person-approach-part-1/

- Learn three ways to control breathing during Pilates https://us.humankinetics.com/blogs/excerpt/learn-three-ways-to-control-breathing-during-pilates

- Pushing Past the Plateau - 3 Easy Ways ... - The Pilates Project https://www.thepilatesproject.net/blog/pushing-past-the-plateau-3-easy-ways-to-go-from-plateau-to-progress-in-pilates

- 13 Impressive Benefits of Pilates, Backed By Science https://www.livestrong.com/article/13778106-benefits-of-pilates/

- 12 Therapist-Backed Tips For Overcoming Exercise Anxiety https://www.huffpost.com/entry/therapist-backed-tips-exercise-anxiety_l_5efb48f8c5b612083c53256c

- Pilates, Mindfulness and Somatic Education - PMC https://www.ncbi.nlm.nih.gov/pmc/articles/PMC4198945/

- 5 Simple Moves That Combine Pilates and HIIT to Transform Your Entire Body https://www.goodhousekeeping.com/health/fitness/a47123/pilates-hiit-workout/

- Pilates Nutrition: Fueling Your Body For Optimal ... https://pilatesreformersplus.com/blogs/news/pilates-nutrition-fueling-your-body-for-optimal-performance-and-recovery

- Pilates Diet Guide: What To Eat Before And After A ... https://betterme.world/articles/pilates-diet/

- Healthy Eating Plan for Pilates Enthusiasts https://www.pinterest.com/ideas/pilates-eating-plan/901586967832/

- Hydration to Maximize Performance and Recovery https://www.ncbi.nlm.nih.gov/pmc/articles/PMC8336541/

- The Health Benefits of Pilates for Older Adults https://www.healthline.com/health/fitness/pilates-for-seniors

- Pilates For Kids : Benefits, Exercises And Teaching Tips https://www.momjunction.com/articles/benefits-of-pilates-for-kids_00330079/

- Pilates helps build self-esteem in the teen years https://www.infinitypilates.com/news/pilates-helps-build-self-esteem-in-the-teen-years/

- Pilates Exercise Modifications https://www.pilatesanytime.com/blog/beginners/pilates-exercise-modifications

- 19 Pilates Benefits Backed By Science https://www.healthline.com/nutrition/pilates-benefits

- A Pilates Success Story: Weight Loss and Walking a Mile https://www.movewellness.com/pilates-success-stories-carol/

- Overcoming Barriers to Physical Activity https://www.cdc.gov/physicalactivity/basics/adding-pa/barriers.html

- Celebrating small goals and achievements in fitness is ... https://www.stylist.co.uk/fitness-health/workouts/small-fitness-achievements/565563

Customer Research

Manuscript Outline

Introduction

Full Manuscript

www.ingramcontent.com/pod-product-compliance
Lightning Source LLC
Chambersburg PA
CBHW080724260726
48660CB00010B/3679